The Ultimate Guide to Carb Cycling for Beginners

Learn How to Rapidly Lose Weight and Maintain a Healthy Diet

Emily Hart

Contents

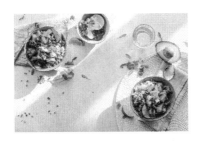

Introduction

If you've ever wondered what Kim Kardashian, Kumail Nanjiani, and Julianne Hough have in common besides their star status, let me clue you in. They've all tapped into the power of carb cycling to achieve their peak physical condition.

Hi there, I'm Emily Hart, and I'm thrilled to be your guide on this journey to understanding and implementing carb cycling. You might be asking, "What exactly is carb cycling, and how can it help me achieve my health and fitness goals?" Well, you're in the right place because we're about to dive deep into this incredibly effective yet often misunderstood dietary strategy.

Carb cycling is a dietary approach that alternates between high-carb and low-carb days to optimize metabolism, promote fat loss, and enhance physical performance when paired with exercise. By strategically manipulating carbohydrate intake, carb cycling leverages the body's natural metabolic processes to achieve remarkable results.

What's truly remarkable about carb cycling is that it's not just a strategy for the rich and famous; it's accessible to anyone looking to transform their body and health. You don't need a personal chef or a bottomless bank account to reap the benefits. With a bit of planning and knowledge, anyone can implement carb cycling, regardless of budget or lifestyle.

One of the most appealing aspects of carb cycling is its flexibility and customization. Unlike rigid diet plans that leave you feeling deprived and restricted, carb cycling allows for individual preferences, goals, and lifestyles. Whether you're a vegetarian, a busy parent, or a hardcore athlete, carb cycling can be tailored to suit your needs. Plus, it's not about cutting out entire food groups or depriving yourself of your favorite treats. Instead, carb cycling emphasizes balance and moderation, making it easier to stick to in the long term while ensuring you're still getting all the essential nutrients your body needs to thrive.

In this comprehensive guide, we'll cover everything you need to know about carb cycling, from the basics of how it works to practical tips for implementing it into your lifestyle. Whether you're looking to shed those stubborn pounds, improve your athletic performance, or simply feel more energized and healthier, carb cycling can help you reach your goals.

Making changes to your diet and lifestyle isn't always easy. Trust me, I've been there. You might be feeling frustrated by previous failed attempts to lose weight or overwhelmed by the sheer volume of conflicting information out there. Maybe you're tired of yo-yo dieting, where you lose a few pounds only to gain them back (plus a few extra) once you return to your old habits. It's enough to make anyone want to throw in the towel and reach for the nearest tub of ice cream.

And let's not even get started on the mental and emotional toll that comes with struggling to achieve your health and fitness goals. The constant self-doubt, the guilt and shame every time you indulge in your favorite foods, and the frustration of seeing other people effortlessly maintain their ideal weight while you're stuck in a never-ending cycle of dieting and deprivation. It's enough to make you want to scream.

But you're not alone, and you're certainly not destined to stay stuck in this cycle forever. I'm here to tell you that there is a better way. Now, I know what you're thinking. "Is carb cycling another diet gimmick? No thanks." But hear me out. Carb cycling isn't some quick-fix solution or magic pill promising overnight results. It's a sustainable, science-backed approach to nutrition that can help you achieve your goals without driving you crazy in the process.

With carb cycling, you won't have to spend hours slaving away on the treadmill or force yourself to choke down tasteless, bland meals. Let's be real: change is never easy, and carb cycling is no exception. You'll face challenges along the way, dealing with cravings, navigating social situations, or simply finding the time and energy to meal prep and exercise. I've been there, I've overcome those challenges, and I'm here to help you do the same.

Growing up in Charleston, SC, I was surrounded by iconic Southern cuisine, which, let's be honest, isn't exactly known for its waistline-friendly dishes. From fried chicken to shrimp and grits, I've indulged in it all.

Like many of you, I've struggled with weight loss since my teenage years. I've tried just about every fad diet out there, from Paleo to Zone to Whole30. And sure, some of them helped me shed a few pounds initially, but I always found myself right back where I started, or worse, a few pounds heavier, once I went off the diet.

That all changed when I discovered carb cycling. This strategic approach to nutrition and exercise helped me lose a whopping 53 lbs. and, more importantly, keep it off for good. Now, I'm here to share everything I've learned with you.

In this book, I'll guide you through the ins and outs of carb cycling, from understanding the science behind it to practical tips for incorporating it into your daily life. Whether you're a carb cycling newbie or a seasoned pro looking to fine-tune your approach, I've got you covered.

I know starting a new diet can be daunting, especially if you've had a few failed attempts in the past. Trust me when I say that carb cycling is different. It's flexible, it's effective, and it's appropriate for everyone, regardless of their age, fitness level, or dietary preferences.

So, if you're ready to say goodbye to crash diets and hello to a sustainable approach to weight loss, you're in the right place. Let's start this journey together and discover how carb cycling can help you achieve your health and fitness goals without compromising your sanity or your lifestyle.

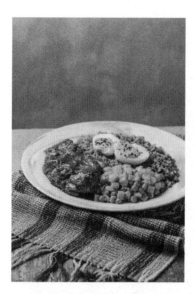

Chapter One

The Fundamentals of Carb Cycling

In this first chapter, we're diving into the nitty-gritty of carb cycling, from understanding how carbohydrates impact metabolism to uncovering the role of insulin in weight management. If you've ever wondered why carbs seem to be the villain in every dieting tale or how they can actually work in your favor, you're about to find out.

Carb cycling isn't just another trendy diet; it's a science-backed approach to nutrition that can revolutionize the way you think about food and fuel your body. We're going to strip away the confusion and get down to the basics, breaking down complex concepts into easy-to-understand nuggets of wisdom. Get ready to discover the incredible benefits of carb cycling, from turbocharging fat loss to skyrocketing your energy levels.

Principles of Carb Cycling: What Is It?

Alright, let's break it down: Carb cycling isn't your typical run-of-the-mill diet plan. It's more like a nutritional strategy that involves playing around with your carb intake on a daily, weekly, or even monthly basis. Picture this: Some days, you're chowing down on pasta like it's going out of style, while on others, you're all about the avocado and eggs. That's the beauty of carb cycling—it's all about flexibility and finding what works best for you. Whether you're fueling up for an intense workout, indulging in a leisurely brunch, or simply satisfying your cravings, carb cycling gives you the freedom to create a menu that nourishes both body and soul.

So, let's dive a little deeper into why we're flipping the script on our carb intake. When you load up on carbs, it's like giving your body a turbo boost of energy to tackle those tough workouts or power through those busy days. You know that feeling when you've just demolished a plate of pasta or polished off a stack of pancakes, and suddenly, you're ready to take on the world? That's the power of carbs in action.

When you dial back on the carbs, a remarkable transformation takes place. Your body, being the incredibly adaptive machine that it is, switches gears and taps into its fat stores for fuel. Yes, you heard that right—by strategically reducing your carb intake, you're essentially training your body to become a fat-burning machine (Zambon, 2021).

I know what you're thinking, "Won't cutting carbs leave me feeling sluggish and hangry?" Trust me, I hear you. It's a common concern and one that's totally valid. After all, carbs have long been touted as our body's preferred source of fuel, so it's natural to worry about what happens when we start cutting back.

Here's the thing, your body is incredibly resilient, and it's more than capable of adapting to changes in your diet. Gradually dialing back on the carbs and incorporating more protein and healthy fats into your meals will leave yourself feeling satisfied and energized, while also giving your body the tools it needs to tap into its fat stores and torch those extra pounds.

Think of carb cycling as a way to have your cake and eat it too—literally. You're still enjoying all the delicious foods you love, but you're doing it in a way that's strategic and purposeful, helping you achieve your health and fitness goals without feeling deprived or restricted. It's the best of both worlds.

Carb cycling isn't just about weight loss; it's also about optimizing your overall health. By cycling between high- and low-carb days, you're giving your body a chance to reap the benefits of both worlds. On high-carb days, you're fueling your muscles and replenishing glycogen stores, while on low-carb days, you're improving insulin sensitivity and burning fat like nobody's business.

You may be thinking, "Emily, isn't eating carbs bad for you?" Not necessarily. You see, not all carbs are created equal. Sure, scarfing down a bag of potato chips might not be the best idea, but loading up on nutrient-dense carbs like fruits, veggies, and whole grains? That's a different story and we'll uncover the reasons why in this book.

The beauty of carb cycling is that it isn't a one-size-fits-all approach. Some people might thrive on a more structured plan, while others prefer a more flexible approach. It's all about finding what works best for you and your body. And hey, if you're not sure where to start, don't worry—I've got your back.

In the next section, we'll dive deeper into science and talk about how carbohydrates can impact your metabolism.

Carbohydrates and Their Impact on Metabolism

Carbohydrates are one of the three main macronutrients in the human diet, alongside protein and fat. These essential molecules, composed of carbon, hydrogen, and oxygen atoms, play a pivotal role in our bodies (Holesh et al., 2023). But let's break down why carbs are so important and how they impact our metabolism.

When we consume carbohydrates, our digestive system goes to work, breaking them down into glucose. Glucose serves as the primary energy source for our cells, fueling everything from our daily activities to intense workouts. Think of carbs as the gas in your car—they keep you moving and performing at your best.

There are two main types of carbohydrates: complex and simple. Understanding the difference between them is key to making smarter dietary choices and keeping your metabolism in check.

First up, we have complex carbohydrates, which include starches and fiber. These carbs are found in foods like whole grains, legumes, and vegetables. What sets complex carbs apart is their chemical structure—they have longer chains of sugar molecules, which means your body takes longer to break them down. This slower digestion process helps prevent blood sugar spikes and keeps your energy levels stable. Plus, complex carbs are packed with essential vitamins, minerals, and fiber, all of which your body needs to function optimally (Cleveland Clinic, 2021).

On the flip side, we have simple carbohydrates, often referred to as sugars. These are found in foods like fruit, milk, and processed snacks. Simple carbs have a much simpler chemical structure, which means your body digests them quickly. While this quick energy boost might sound appealing, it can lead to rapid spikes in blood sugar, followed by crashes. Consuming too many simple carbs can contribute to weight gain and increase your risk of developing diabetes, heart disease, and high cholesterol (Cleveland Clinic, 2021).

The goal is to prioritize complex carbs in your diet for sustained energy and overall health while being mindful of your intake of simple carbs to avoid those unwanted blood sugar rollercoasters. We will cover this topic in greater detail later in this book.

Carb Cycling Impacts on Metabolism

How exactly does carb cycling impact your metabolism? The concept is pretty fascinating and can be a game-changer for those looking to optimize their health and fitness. Let's dive into the mechanics of this approach and see why alternating between high-carb and low-carb days can significantly affect your metabolic function.

At its core, carb cycling is about strategically leveraging the benefits of carbohydrates. On high-carb days, you're essentially fueling your body with the energy it needs for intense physical activity and recovery. Think of these days as giving your body a supercharged boost—you're loading up on carbs to replenish glycogen stores, which are the primary energy source for your muscles during exercise. This influx of energy helps enhance your performance, allowing you to push harder during workouts.

There's more to it than just performance enhancement, consuming more carbs on these days also triggers what's known as the thermic effect of food (TEF). TEF is the amount of energy your body uses to digest, absorb, and process the nutrients in your food. Carbohydrates have a relatively high thermic effect, meaning your metabolism revs up to handle the increased intake (Reed & Hill, 1996). This can lead to a temporary boost in your metabolic rate, helping you burn more calories even when you're not working out.

Now, let's talk about the low-carb days. When you reduce your carbohydrate intake, your body has to find an alternative energy source to keep you going. Enter fat metabolism. On these days, your body switches gears and starts to burn stored fat for fuel. The metabolic shift not only aids in fat loss but also promotes more efficient metabolic function over time.

The main appeal of carb cycling lies in its adaptability. By alternating between high- and low-carb days, you're essentially keeping your metabolism on its toes. Variability in your diet helps prevent the metabolic slowdown that often accompanies long-term dieting or extreme calorie restriction. Your body becomes more flexible in switching between different energy sources, which can lead to better overall metabolic health.

Let's put this into perspective with an example. Imagine you've planned a high-intensity workout for Monday. On this day, you increase your carb intake, focusing on nutrient-dense sources like sweet potatoes, quinoa, and fruits. Your body will use these carbs to power through your workout, enhancing performance and aiding in muscle recovery. The TEF kicks in, resulting in your metabolism receiving a nice little boost.

Come Tuesday, it's a rest day or a lighter workout. You switch to a low-carb approach, focusing more on proteins and healthy fats—think eggs, avocado, and leafy greens. With fewer carbs available, your body turns to its fat stores for energy. This shift not only helps with burning fat but also keeps your metabolism active and engaged.

Alternating this pattern creates a metabolic environment that's dynamic and responsive. High-carb days prevent your metabolism from getting too sluggish, while low-carb days promote fat-burning and metabolic efficiency. It's a balanced approach that aligns with your body's natural rhythms and energy needs.

The Role of Insulin in Weight Management

Insulin is a critical player in the weight management game, this hormone does so much more than just regulate blood sugar levels. It's a key influence on how our body handles carbs, burns fat, stores fat, and even how hungry we feel. Understanding insulin's role can be a game-changer in your weight loss journey.

Influences your Metabolism: Your body breaks carbohydrates down into glucose, which enters your bloodstream. This increase in blood sugar triggers your pancreas to release insulin. Think of insulin as a traffic cop directing glucose into your cells, where it's used for energy. Insulin's role doesn't just stop there, it also signals your liver to store any excess glucose as glycogen for later use.

Due to its high thermic effect, insulin causes your body to burn more calories processing carbs when its levels are higher. This can temporarily boost your metabolism, which is one of the reasons why high-carb days in carb cycling can be beneficial. Alternating high-low carb days helps to keep your metabolic rate from slowing down, a common issue with strict, long-term dieting.

Metabolic Adaptation: Now, let's touch on metabolic adaptation, your body's ability to adjust its metabolism based on your dietary intake and energy expenditure. Consistently consuming a high-carb diet makes your body efficient at using glucose for energy. Over time, however, this can result in insulin resistance, where your cells become less responsive to insulin's signals. Weight loss can then become more difficult and elevate the risk of developing type 2 diabetes.

Incorporating low-carb days through carb cycling can help prevent metabolic adaptation. Low-carb days enhance insulin sensitivity, allowing your body to respond more effectively to insulin. Enhanced insulin sensitivity can boost your overall metabolic health and support long-term weight management.

Affects Fat Burning: When you reduce your carb intake, your insulin levels drop. Lower insulin levels signal your body to start burning fat for fuel instead of relying on glucose. This is one of the reasons why low-carb diets and carb cycling are effective for fat loss.

When insulin levels are low, your body's fat-burning machinery kicks into high gear. Your body becomes more efficient at breaking down stored fat, turning them into fatty acids, which can then be used for energy. Metabolic flexibility is key to effective weight management and is one of the major benefits of incorporating low-carb days into your diet.

Drives Fat Storage: Insulin is also known as the "fat-storing hormone." When insulin levels are high, your body is in storage mode. Any excess glucose that isn't used for energy or stored as glycogen gets converted into fat. This process is called lipogenesis, and it's your body's way of ensuring it has a backup energy reserve (Nesterova et al., 2020).

Consistently high insulin levels, often due to a diet high in refined sugars and carbs, can lead to increased fat storage, which over time, can result in weight gain, particularly around the midsection. Managing your carb intake and keeping insulin levels in check are crucial for preventing unwanted fat accumulation.

Impacts Appetite: In addition to influencing the way your body handles carbs and fats, insulin also plays a significant role in appetite regulation. When you eat a meal high in carbs, your blood sugar temporarily spikes, followed by a temporary spike in insulin before these levels fall back down. The rapid rise and fall can lead to hunger pangs and cravings shortly after eating, resembling a rollercoaster for your appetite.

Conversely, a low-carb meals can help stabilize blood sugar and insulin levels, leading to more consistent energy levels and reduced hunger. Stabilizing your insulin levels makes you less likely to experience intense cravings for sugary or high-carb foods which can help you stick to your dietary goals and avoid overeating.

Putting It All Together

How can you manage insulin levels effectively to support weight loss? Here are some tips:

•**Adopt a low-carb diet:** Incorporate low-carb days into your weekly routine to help lower insulin levels and promote fat burning. Focus on whole foods like lean proteins, healthy fats, and plenty of vegetables.

•**Choose complex carbs:** When you consume carbs, opt for complex carbs like whole grains, legumes, and fiber-rich vegetables. These carbs have a lower glycemic index, meaning they cause a slower, more gradual rise in blood sugar and insulin levels.

•**Monitor portions:** Even with healthy carbs, portion control is key. Too much of any macronutrient can lead to excess calorie intake and potential weight gain.

•**Stay active:** Regular physical activity helps improve insulin sensitivity and supports overall metabolic health. Aim for a mix of cardio and strength-training exercises.

•**Stay hydrated:** Drinking plenty of water can help regulate appetite and support your metabolism.

•**Get enough sleep:** Poor sleep can negatively affect insulin sensitivity and increase hunger hormones. Aim for 7-9 hours of quality sleep each night.

•**Manage stress:** Chronic stress can lead to elevated cortisol levels, which can negatively impact insulin sensitivity. Incorporate stress-reducing activities like meditation, yoga, or deep breathing exercises into your routine.

Benefits of Carb Cycling

The carb cycling approach isn't just about eating carbs one day and cutting them the next; it's a strategic way to optimize your health, performance, and weight management. Let's break down the various advantages and how carb cycling can be a game-changer for you.

Improved Energy: Ever feel like you hit a wall during your workouts or by mid-afternoon? Carb cycling can help with that. On high-carb days, you're fueling your body with glycogen, which is your muscles' primary energy source. For those who are very active, this fuel is especially crucial. When you have ample glycogen stores, you can perform better during intense workouts, whether it's a marathon, martial arts, or a Tough Mudder challenge. High-carb days ensure you have the energy to power through those demanding activities and recover faster afterward.

Flipping to low-carb days, these help your body become more efficient at burning fat for fuel. Gaining metabolic flexibility means you can maintain steady energy levels even when you're not consuming a lot of carbs. The result? You avoid the dreaded energy crashes that come with a high-sugar diet and stay energized throughout the day.

Lose Fat or Weight – Gain Muscle: Carb cycling can be incredibly effective for shedding fat while preserving or even building muscle. When carb consumption is reduced, your body switches to burning fat for fuel, which helps with weight loss. Periods of reduced carb intake can enhance insulin sensitivity, making your body more efficient at using carbs when you do consume them, further supporting fat loss.

It's not just about losing fat through carb cycling though. Carbohydrates are crucial for muscle gain. Carbs stimulate the release of insulin, which acts as a growth-promoting hormone that aids in muscle repair and growth. This is why bodybuilders and athletes often see better muscle gains on a higher-carb diet. Cycling between high- and low-carb optimizes both fat loss and muscle gain, getting the best of both worlds.

You Get to Eat Carbs! One of the most appealing aspects of carb cycling is that you don't have to give up carbs entirely. Unlike strict low-carb or keto diets, carb cycling allows you to enjoy your favorite carb-rich foods regularly. Having flexibility makes it much easier to stick to your diet long-term because you're not constantly feeling deprived.

Imagine being able to enjoy a delicious pasta dish or a sweet potato without guilt. You can indulge in these foods on high-carb days, knowing they're part of your plan. Carb cycling allows you to enjoy social situations, dining out, and family meals without added stress from dietary restrictions.

Better Performance and Recovery: For those who are active or athletic, carb cycling offers a way to enhance performance and recovery. With low-carb or keto diets, your body relies on fat and stored glycogen for fuel. However, during intense and prolonged physical activities, glycogen stores can become depleted, leading to fatigue and decreased performance. Carb cycling allows you to refill your glycogen stores on high-carb days, ensuring better performance and quicker recovery in subsequent workouts.

Whether you're lifting weights, running marathons, or engaging in high-intensity interval training, having the right fuel at the right time can make a significant difference in your performance and how quickly you bounce back.

Break Through Plateaus: Hitting a weight-loss plateau can be incredibly frustrating. If you've been following a low-carb or keto diet and your progress has stalled, carb cycling might be the solution. Implementing high-carb days can stimulate leptin production, boosting your metabolism and promoting fat loss, which helps you break through stubborn plateaus and continue making progress toward your goals.

Support Gut Health: One often overlooked aspect of strict low-carb diets is their potential impact on gut health. Getting enough fiber on a low-carb or keto diet can be challenging and can affect the health of your gut microbiome. Carb cycling unlocks a wider variety of foods, including high-fiber options like potatoes, yams, carrots, and beets. These foods provide essential fiber that fuels your gut microbes, helping them produce beneficial compounds like butyrate, which has anti-inflammatory properties.

Maintaining a healthy gut is crucial for overall well-being, and carb cycling can help you achieve a more balanced diet that supports digestive health.

More Dietary Flexibility: Carb cycling also provides greater dietary flexibility, offering a welcome relief for those who feel constrained by strict low-carb or keto diets. It allows you to enjoy a wider variety of foods and reduces the stress associated with rigid eating patterns. Whether you're dining out with friends, enjoying a special meal at home, or simply navigating the grocery store, carb cycling gives you the freedom to include more of the foods you love.

Reducing stress around food can have significant benefits for your mental and emotional well-being. Dieting shouldn't feel like a constant battle, and carb cycling offers a way to enjoy your meals while still working toward your health and fitness goals.

Low Carb Benefits: Low-carb days bring their own set of benefits, particularly for metabolic health. Lowering carb intake can greatly improve insulin sensitivity, enabling your body to manage blood sugar levels more effectively. Improving insulin sensitivity is vital for preventing and managing conditions such as type 2 diabetes.

Periods of lower carb intake also boost fat burning. With fewer carbs available, your body taps into fat stores for energy, promoting weight loss. Additionally, low-carb diets are known to improve cholesterol levels by increasing HDL (the good cholesterol) and reducing LDL (the bad cholesterol) in some individuals, potentially lowering your risk of heart disease and supporting your overall metabolic health.

Alternating between low and high-carb days allows you to enjoy the benefits of both approaches without the downsides of sticking to one extreme.

High Carb Advantages: High-carb days have great benefits too! Refeeding with carbs can positively impact several key hormones, such as thyroid hormones, testosterone, and leptin. Hormones like these are crucial for regulating hunger, metabolism, and exercise performance.

Thyroid hormones play a significant role in your metabolic rate. High-carb days can help keep these hormones at optimal levels, preventing the metabolic slowdown that often accompanies prolonged low-carb dieting. Testosterone is vital for muscle growth and recovery, and higher carb intake supports its production.

Leptin, often referred to as the "satiety hormone," helps regulate your appetite (Gunnars, 2018). When you consume carbs, leptin levels increase, which can help reduce hunger and make it easier to stick to your dietary goals. High-carb intervals can also reduce inflammation and improve iron utilization, both of which are important for overall health and recovery.

So, if you're looking for a sustainable and effective approach to nutrition, carb cycling might just be the answer you've been searching for.

I want to take a moment to recognize the process that you are about to start. I know how daunting it can be to start yet another eating regime, especially after the fact that you may have struggled with weight throughout your life. I know; I have been there.

Dieting is an industry full of confusion, broken promises, and fads. The truth is, carb cycling is no fad, it is the most strategic nutritional lifestyle that will allow you to regain control over your health and yield results that will actually stick.

I know how aggravating it is to try out many diets that don't work, only to end up right back where you began. I've been on both sides of the fence with relative initial success, only to later see the pounds creep back on. That road is one I've traveled more times than I care to admit. And here I am today, to take you through the basics of carb cycling, with my experience and story echoing in and out. We shall feel the highs and lows of the journey, celebrate the victories, and learn from the failures.

As we begin this journey, I want you to be empowered and excited about what you have in front of you. We are not discussing just another diet plan here; we are discussing a lifestyle transformation that can completely reshape not only your body but your mindset when it comes to food and exercise. So, breathe that sigh of relief, have some confidence in the process, and realize you are not on this ride alone.

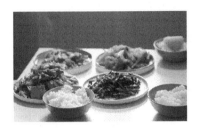

Chapter Two

The Carb Cycling Blueprint—Let's Get Started

If you're eager to learn how to implement carb cycling into your daily life and start seeing real results, you're in the right place. In this chapter, we'll walk through the step-by-step process of getting started with carb cycling. From calculating your macronutrient needs to creating a customized plan that fits your lifestyle and goals, we've got you covered.

Starting something new can feel overwhelming, but don't worry—I'm here to guide you every step of the way. Together, we'll break down the key concepts and set you up for success on your carb cycling journey.

Get Started by Understanding Macronutrients and Basal Metabolic Rate

Before we jump into the plan itself, we need to understand the basics of macronutrients and how our body uses energy. This knowledge will be your foundation for crafting an effective and personalized carb cycling strategy.

Macronutrients are the cornerstone of your diet, they're the nutrients your body needs in large amounts for energy and proper functioning. There are three main types: carbohydrates, proteins, and fats. Each plays a unique role in your body, and getting the right balance is crucial for success in carb cycling.

Carbohydrates are your body's go-to fuel source, playing a crucial role in maintaining your overall health and vitality. As we've discussed, when you consume carbs, your body breaks them down into glucose, a simple sugar that serves as the primary energy source for your brain, muscles, and other vital functions. Glucose circulates in your bloodstream and is transported to your cells, where it's either used immediately for energy or stored for later use (Pearson, 2017).

In the context of carb cycling, carbs are especially important on high-carb days, when you're gearing up for intense workouts or need to recover from strenuous physical activity. Loading up on carbs will ensure that your muscles have enough glycogen (stored glucose) to power through those tough sessions. Not only does this enhance your performance, but it also aids in quicker recovery, allowing your muscles to repair and grow more efficiently.

Carbohydrates are found in a wide variety of foods, including grains, fruits, vegetables, and legumes. It's important to note, not all carbs are created equal. We've already touched on the two main types of carbohydrates—complex and simple—in the previous chapter. Now, let's break them down further:

Complex carbohydrates are found in whole grains, vegetables, legumes, and some fruits. They have longer chains of sugar molecules, meaning they take longer to digest. A slower digestion process provides a steady release of glucose into your bloodstream, offering sustained energy and preventing the spikes and crashes associated with simple carbs. A key benefit of complex carbs is their fiber content. Fiber is a type of carbohydrate that your body can't digest, which means it doesn't contribute calories, but it plays a vital role in digestive health. Fiber helps regulate blood sugar levels, aids in digestion, and keeps you feeling full longer, making it an essential component of a balanced diet (Cherney, 2023). Foods rich in complex carbohydrates include:

Whole grains: Brown rice, quinoa, oatmeal, and whole wheat bread
Vegetables: Sweet potatoes, broccoli, spinach, and carrots
Legumes: Lentils, chickpeas, black beans, and peas

Simple carbohydrates are composed of shorter chains of sugar molecules. They're found in foods like fruits, milk, and processed items like candies and soft drinks. These carbs are digested quickly, leading to rapid spikes in blood sugar and insulin levels. Simple carbs can provide a quick burst of energy, but they often lead to energy crashes, making you feel tired and hungry shortly after eating. While some simple carbs, like those found in fruits and milk, come with essential vitamins and minerals, others, particularly those in processed foods, offer little nutritional value and are often linked to weight gain and health issues like type 2 diabetes and heart disease (Cherney, 2023). Examples of foods high in simple carbohydrates include:

Refined grains: White bread, pasta, and pastries
Sugary snacks: Candies, cookies, and cakes
Sugary drinks: Soda, fruit juices, and energy drinks

Proteins play a multifaceted role in your overall health, from repairing tissues to fueling muscle growth and supporting immune function. Proteins step into the spotlight, especially on low-carb days, as they provide crucial support for muscle maintenance and growth while keeping hunger at bay.

Every day, your body undergoes a continuous cycle of wear and tear. Whether it's the microscopic tears in your muscles after a workout or the daily cellular turnover in your organs, protein is there to pick up the pieces and set the stage for regeneration. Without an adequate supply of protein, your body would struggle to repair tissues, leading to slower recovery times and an increased risk of injury (Van De Walle, 2023).

If you're aiming to shed excess pounds and sculpt a lean physique, protein is your best friend. Not only does it help preserve existing muscle mass during periods of calorie restriction, it also fuels the growth of new muscle tissue when paired with strength training. On low-carb days, when your body relies on stored fat for fuel, adequate protein intake is particularly important to ensure your muscles remain strong and resilient.

Fortunately, there's no shortage of delicious and nutritious sources of protein to choose from. Whether you prefer animal-based options or plant-based alternatives, there's something to suit every palate and dietary preference. Good sources of protein include:

Lean meats: Chicken breast, turkey, lean cuts of beef, and pork loin

Fish: Salmon, tuna, trout, and cod are not only rich in protein but also packed with heart-healthy omega-3 fatty acids

Eggs: A versatile and affordable protein source, eggs are nutrient powerhouses, providing a complete array of essential amino acids

Dairy products: Greek yogurt, cottage cheese, and low-fat milk offer a convenient way to boost your protein intake while also providing bone-strengthening calcium

Legumes: Beans, lentils, and chickpeas are excellent plant-based sources of protein, as well as fiber and essential nutrients

Nuts and seeds: Almonds, walnuts, chia seeds, and hemp seeds are protein-rich but also brimming with healthy fats and antioxidants

Fats are essential for energy, hormone production, and nutrient absorption while also helping to keep you feeling full and satisfied. In carb cycling, fats become more prominent on low-carb days, providing a steady energy source when carbs are limited.

Healthy fats are found in foods like avocados, nuts, seeds, olive oil, and fatty fish. These fats support heart health and overall well-being, making them a crucial part of your diet (Harvard Health Publishing, 2021).

Converting Macronutrients into Calories

Understanding how to convert macronutrients into calories is essential for managing your intake. Here's a quick breakdown (Kubala, 2018):

1 gram of carbohydrates = 4 calories
1 gram of protein = 4 calories
1 gram of fat = 9 calories

This information helps you calculate your daily calorie intake based on the macronutrient composition of your meals. For instance, if you consume 50 grams of carbs, 30 grams of protein, and 20 grams of fat in a meal, you can calculate the total calories as follows:

Carbs: 50g x 4 = 200 calories
Protein: 30g x 4 = 120 calories
Fat: 20g x 9 = 180 calories
Total = 500 calories

By understanding these conversions, you can tailor your diet to meet your specific caloric and macronutrient needs, which are essential for effective carb cycling.

Basal Metabolic Rate (BMR)

Your Basal Metabolic Rate (BMR) is the number of calories your body needs to maintain basic physiological functions while at rest, such as breathing, circulation, and cell production. It's the minimum energy requirement for your body to function (Garnet Health, 2016).

To calculate your BMR you can use various formulas such as the Harris-Benedict formula, however, we will use the Mifflin-St. Jeor equation in this book.

Alternatively, you can use online BMR calculators for a quick and easy estimate. Knowing your BMR is crucial because it gives you a baseline for the minimum calories you need to support your body's essential functions.

Total Daily Energy Expenditure (TDEE)

While BMR provides a baseline, it's not the whole picture. Your Total Daily Energy Expenditure (TDEE) includes all the calories you burn in a day, factoring in your physical activity levels. TDEE is a more comprehensive measure of your daily calorie needs and is essential for creating an effective diet plan (Phelps, 2019).

TDEE = BMR + (calories burned through physical activity)

To calculate your TDEE, you need to consider your activity level, which can range from sedentary to very active. Here's a quick guide to help you determine your activity level (Phelps, 2019):

Sedentary (little to no exercise): BMR x 1.2

Lightly active (light exercise/sports 1–3 days/week): BMR x 1.375

Moderately active (moderate exercise/sports 3–5 days/week): BMR x 1.55

Very active (hard exercise or sports 6–7 days a week): BMR x 1.725

Super active (very hard exercise/sports & physical job): BMR x 1.9

For example, if your BMR is 1500 calories and you are moderately active, your TDEE would be:

TDEE = 1500 x 1.55 = 2325 calories

This means you need 2325 calories per day to maintain your current weight with your activity level.

Calculating Your Carb Cycling Plan

Alright, let's dive into the details of setting up your carb cycling plan. To get started, we'll need to crunch some numbers to determine your Basal Metabolic Rate (BMR), Total Daily Energy Expenditure (TDEE), and macronutrient ratios. Don't worry; I'll walk you through each step, and we'll have you carb-cycling like a pro in no time!

Step 1: Calculate Your BMR

We'll use the Mifflin-St Jeor Equation, a widely accepted formula for estimating BMR based on age, gender, weight, and height (Mifflin-St Jeor Equation, 2020).

Mifflin-St Jeor Equation:
For Men: BMR = (10 × weight in kg) + (6.25 × height in cm) - (5 × age in years) + 5

For Women: BMR = (10 × weight in kg) + (6.25 × height in cm) - (5 × age in years) - 161

Let's put this into practice with an example. Suppose you're a 30-year-old woman who weighs 70 kg and is 165 cm tall:

BMR = (10 x 70) + (6.25 x 165) - (5 x 30) - 161
BMR = 700 + 1031.25 - 150 -161
BMR = 1420.25

Your BMR would be approximately 1420 calories per day.

Once you've calculated your BMR, we'll move on to the next step.

Step 2: Determine Your TDEE

Your Total Daily Energy Expenditure (TDEE) takes into account your activity level on top of your BMR. This is the total number of calories your body needs to maintain your current weight, factoring in physical activity and exercise.

To calculate your TDEE, simply multiply your BMR by your Physical Activity Level (PAL), which ranges from sedentary (little to no exercise) to very active (intense exercise or physical job). For reference, you can find the values previously mentioned in this chapter.

Using our example, let's say you are moderately active:

$$TDEE = BMR \times 1.55$$
$$TDEE = 1420.25 \times 1.55$$
$$TDEE = 2201.39$$

So, your TDEE would be approximately 2201 calories per day.

Step 3: Calculate Your Macronutrient Ratios

Now that we have your TDEE, it's time to determine the ideal macronutrient ratios for your carb cycling plan. For weight loss, we typically aim for the following ratios:

Carbohydrates: 10-30%
Protein: 40-50%
Fat: 30-40%

These ratios provide a balanced approach to fueling your body while promoting fat loss and muscle maintenance.

Step 4: Convert Macros into Daily Calories

To translate these ratios into practical terms, we'll convert them into daily calorie targets for each macronutrient. Remember, each gram of carbohydrate and protein provides 4 calories, while each gram of fat provides 9 calories.

Here's how to calculate your daily intake for each macronutrient:

Daily carbohydrate intake: TDEE × (10–30%) / 4
Daily protein intake: TDEE × (40–50%) / 4
Daily fat intake: TDEE × (30–40%) / 9

Now, let's put it all together with an example to make things crystal clear. Let's say your calculated TDEE is 2000 calories per day. Using the recommended macronutrient ratios:

Carbohydrates: 20% of 2000 calories = 400 calories / 4 = 100 g
Protein: 45% of 2000 calories = 900 calories / 4 = 225 g
Fat: 35% of 2000 calories = 700 calories / 9 = 78 g

Based on these calculations, your daily macronutrient targets would be approximately 100 g of carbohydrates, 225 g of protein, and 78 g of fat.

By following these steps and tailoring your macronutrient intake to your specific needs and goals, you'll be well-equipped to embark on your carb cycling journey with confidence.

What Your Food Intake Looks Like on High-Carb vs Low-Carb Days

Alright, let's get into the juicy details of what you'll actually be eating on high-carb and low-carb days. This is where the rubber meets the road in carb cycling, and it's all about understanding how to balance your macros to match your activity levels and goals.

The typical macro ratios you'll be aiming for on high-carb and low-carb days are as follows:

Low-Carb Days
- 10% Carbohydrates
- 50% Protein
- 40% Fat

High-Carb Days
- 30% Carbohydrates
- 50% Protein
- 20% Fat

Notice something important here: On high-carb days, you'll be consuming less fat, and on low-carb days, you'll be consuming more fat.Ensuring this balance gives your body the necessary fuel to function optimally,whether you're pushing through an intense workout or allowing your body to restand recover.

What Does a High-Carb Day Look Like?

High-carb days focus on loading up on carbs to fuel your workouts and aid in recovery, providing the extra energy your body needs to perform at its best during intense physical activities. By aligning these days with more demanding exercise sessions, you ensure your body has the necessary resources to optimize performance and support recovery.

For a high-carb day example, you're planning a tough weightlifting session followed by a long run. Here's how you might structure your meals:

> ### Breakfast
> A big bowl of oatmeal topped with berries, a spoonful of almond butter, and a drizzle of honey with a protein shake inclusive of a scoop of protein powder, a banana, and a handful of spinach
> ### Snack
> Greek yogurt with granola and sliced fruit
> ### Lunch
> Grilled chicken breast with a quinoa salad loaded with veggies like cherry tomatoes, cucumbers, and bell peppers with a side of sweet potato fries
> ### Snack
> An apple with a handful of almonds
> ### Dinner
> Baked salmon with a side of brown rice and steamed broccoli with a mixed green salad tossed in a light vinaigrette
> ### Post-Workout Snack
> A protein smoothie with a scoop of protein powder, frozen berries, and a splash of almond milk

What Does a Low-Carb Day Look Like?

Low-carb days are designed to help your body tap into its fat stores for energy, making them ideal for lighter activity or rest days. On these days, a higher fat intake helps keep you satiated, while adequate protein supports muscle repair and maintenance, ensuring your body remains fueled and your muscles stay strong even during periods of reduced physical activity.

Here's an example of a low-carb day where you might be focusing on recovery with some light stretching or yoga:

Breakfast
An omelet with spinach, mushrooms, and cheese, cooked in olive oil with a side of avocado slices

Snack
Celery sticks with almond butter

Lunch
Grilled chicken Caesar salad with plenty of leafy greens, cherry tomatoes, and a generous helping of avocado along with a handful of mixed nuts

Snack
A hard-boiled egg with a few slices of turkey breast

Dinner
Beef stir-fry with lots of veggies like bell peppers, broccoli, and zucchini, cooked in coconut oil with a side of cauliflower rice

Evening Snack
A small bowl of cottage cheese with a sprinkle of chia seeds

To really nail your carb cycling plan, it's crucial to keep track of your macros and adjust as needed. Using apps like MyFitnessPal or Cronometer can be incredibly helpful for logging your food intake and ensuring you're hitting your targets.

Let me share a quick anecdote. When I first started carb cycling, I was a bit overwhelmed by all the calculations and planning, but once I got the hang of it, I noticed a significant boost in my energy levels on high-carb days and better fat loss on low-carb days. One of my favorite high-carb meals is a hearty quinoa and black bean salad with lots of veggies and a zesty lime dressing. On low-carb days, I love whipping up a creamy avocado and chicken salad that keeps me full and satisfied.

Understanding the balance between high-carb and low-carb days is crucial for making carb cycling work for you. Carefully planning your meals and focusing on macronutrient ratios can optimize energy levels, support muscle growth, and promote fat loss. Remember, high-carb days are all about fueling performance, while low-carb days focus on burning fat and maintaining muscle.

We've covered a lot so far, haven't we? You now have all the essential tools to begin your journey into the world of carb cycling. But let's be honest for a moment here — launching something new can be a pretty terrifying thing, and I can completely respect that.

I was very excited and nervous when I first began carb cycling — I was so eager and full of anticipation that I'd get in my own way, worrying if I could really do it and skeptical if it would actually work. While it wasn't a perfectly smooth transition, I learned the most important thing was to just have patience with myself and keep on keeping on. I had days where I nailed my macros and felt like I was on top of the world and could conquer it, and ones where I messed up and got a little uptight. And that's fine — progress isn't always perfect.

I want you to know that it is all right to struggle and to be doubtful. We are all in it together, and all of us must keep in mind that every single step that you take may be small, but it is one in the right direction. Be gentle with yourself and keep fine-tuning your plan until it fits like a glove into your life.

As we continue on, we're going to start to get into the nuts and bolts of really fine-tuning your nutrition plan for quite literally the best results possible. Consider this next chapter as an extension of carb cycling, you've learned the basics, and now you can fine-tune and tailor your own plan.

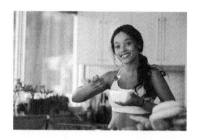

Chapter Three

Fine-Tuning Your Nutritional Plan for Enhanced Results

Are you ready to kick your carb cycling program up a notch? This chapter will be your master plan for making everything you eat work harder for you.

Nutrient Timing

One of the most impactful aspects of carb cycling is the strategic timing of nutrient intake. What you eat greatly affects your workout performance and recovery, so it's crucial to get it right for carb cycling success. Understanding and implementing the best eating practices can elevate your results from good to phenomenal. Mastering nutrient timing can significantly enhance your overall fitness journey.

Consuming the right nutrients before and after your workouts is essential. It's not just about what you eat; when you eat it, can make a huge difference in how you feel and perform as well. Here are some of the best practice strategies for pre- and post- workout nutrition.

Pre-Workout Nutrition

3–4 Hours Before Exercise: Eat a Full Meal. To maximize your workout efforts, it's important to eat a full meal about 3–4 hours before exercising. This meal should be balanced, containing a good mix of carbohydrates, protein, and fats. The carbs will provide the necessary fuel, the protein will help support muscle maintenance, and the fats will offer sustained energy.

Here's an example of what this meal could look like:

> **Carbs:** Quinoa or brown rice
> **Protein:** Grilled chicken or tofu
> **Fats:** Avocado or olive oil
> **Veggies:** A generous serving of your favorite vegetables

A combination such as this ensures that you have a steady stream of energy throughout your workout and that your muscles are primed and ready to go.

1–2 Hours Before Exercise: Consume a High-Carb Snack. About one to two hours before you hit the gym, it's beneficial to have a higher-carb snack, especially if you're on a high-carb day, as it gives you that quick boost of energy needed for intense workouts. Think of something light but packed with easily digestible carbs.

Some great options include:

> • A banana with a spoonful of almond butter
> • A smoothie with a scoop of protein powder, a handful of berries, and a splash of almond milk
> • A slice of whole-grain toast with honey

These snacks will ensure that your glycogen stores are topped up, giving you the energy to power through your session without feeling sluggish.

Post-Workout Nutrition

Within 2 Hours Post-Workout: Consume a Meal. After your workout, your body is like a sponge, ready to soak up nutrients to repair and build muscle. Aim to eat a balanced meal within two hours after your workout, incorporating both carbohydrates and protein. Consuming carbohydrates helps replenish your glycogen stores, while the protein provides the amino acids essential for muscle repair and growth. This combination optimizes recovery and enhances the benefits of your training session.

Here's an example of a post-workout meal:

Carbs: Sweet potato or whole-grain pasta
Protein: Salmon or a plant-based protein source like lentils
Veggies: A variety of colorful vegetables for added nutrients

2–3 Hours Before Bed Stop Eating. It's generally best to stop eating 2-3 hours before bedtime as your body needs to wind down and prepare for restful sleep without an overactive digestive system. If you're really hungry, a light evening snack is fine, but heavy meals should be avoided late at night.

Pre-Workout Nutrition Benefits

Energy boost: Eating before exercise gives you the fuel needed to perform at your best. Carbs are your body's primary energy source and having them in your system ensures that you can tackle your workout with vigor.

Enhanced performance: A well-fueled body means you can push harder and go longer during your workouts. This leads to better performance and more effective sessions, whether you're lifting weights, running, or engaging in high-intensity interval training.

Prevents fatigue: Starting your workout with a full tank of energy helps prevent early fatigue, allowing you to maintain intensity and focus throughout your exercise routine.

Post-Workout Benefits

Muscle repair: After exercise, your muscles need protein to repair and grow. Consuming protein post-workout provides the essential amino acids necessary for this process, reducing muscle soreness and enhancing recovery.

Reduced muscle soreness: Proper post-workout nutrition can help minimize muscle soreness and stiffness, making it easier to stay consistent with your workout routine.

Glycogen replenishment: Carbs post-workout help replenish glycogen stores depleted during exercise. This is crucial for recovery, especially if you have another workout planned within the next 24 hours.

Optimized recovery: The right balance of carbs and protein post-workout ensures that your body recovers efficiently, preparing you for your next training session and helping you progress toward your fitness goals.

Here are some ways to implement these nutrient timing strategies into your daily life.

• **Meal prep:** One of the best ways to ensure you're getting the right nutrients at the right times is to plan and prep your meals ahead of time. Spend a couple of hours each week preparing meals and snacks that align with your workout schedule. This way, you'll always have the right foods on hand, making it easier to stick to your plan.

• **Listen to your body:** Pay attention to how your body feels with different timing strategies. Everyone is different, and what works for one person might not work for another. If you find that eating a full meal

3 hours before a workout leaves you feeling sluggish, try adjusting the timing or portion size until you find what works best for you.

• **Stay hydrated:** Don't forget about hydration! Drinking plenty of water before, during, and after your workouts is crucial for maintaining energy levels and supporting recovery. Consider adding a pinch of sea salt to your water to help with electrolyte balance, especially if you're engaging in long or intense workouts.

• **Quality over quantity:** Focus on the quality of your foods rather than just the quantity. Choose whole, nutrient-dense foods that provide sustained energy and essential nutrients. Avoid processed foods that can cause energy crashes and hinder your performance and recovery.

Nutrient timing is a powerful tool in your carb cycling toolkit. Plan your meals and snacks around your workouts to boost performance, speed up recovery, and get the most out of your training. It's all about figuring out what works best for you and making small adjustments along the way. Having a personalized approach helps your nutrition support your fitness goals, improving both your performance and overall well-being.

How Your Body Utilizes Carbs

One of the most essential topics when it comes to carb cycling is understanding how your body utilizes carbohydrates. It might sound a bit technical, but don't worry—I'm here to break it down in a way that's easy to understand.

When you eat foods that contain carbohydrates, your body undergoes a fascinating series of processes to convert these carbs into usable energy. Let's walk through this journey step by step.

Step 1: Digestion Begins in the Mouth

The moment you take a bite of a carb-rich food, like a slice of bread or an apple, the digestion process kicks off in your mouth. Your saliva contains an enzyme called amylase, which starts breaking down complex carbohydrates into simpler sugars. This is the first step in turning the food you eat into energy.

Step 2: Breaking Down in the Stomach and Small Intestine

Once you swallow, the food travels down your esophagus and lands in your stomach, where it's mixed with stomach acids. These acids help break down the food further, preparing it for the next stage of digestion in the small intestine.

In the small intestine, enzymes continue to work on breaking down carbohydrates. Here, complex carbs are broken down into simple sugars, primarily glucose. This process is crucial because your body can only absorb simple sugars into the bloodstream.

Step 3: Absorption into the Bloodstream

As the simple sugars are broken down, they're absorbed through the walls of the small intestine and into your bloodstream. This is where glucose comes into play. Glucose is the primary sugar that your body uses for energy, and once it enters the bloodstream, it's transported to various cells throughout your body.

Step 4: The Role of Insulin

When glucose enters your bloodstream, your blood sugar levels rise and in response to this, your pancreas releases a hormone called insulin. Insulin acts as a key that unlocks cells, allowing glucose to enter and be used for energy.

Think of insulin as a traffic director, guiding glucose to where it's needed most. It ensures that your muscles, brain, and other vital organs receive the energy they need to function properly. Without insulin, glucose would remain in the bloodstream, leading to elevated blood sugar levels.

Step 5: Energy Production

Once inside the cells, glucose undergoes a process called glycolysis, where it's broken down further to produce adenosine triphosphate (ATP). ATP is the energy currency of your cells, providing the power needed for everything from muscle contractions during a workout to maintaining basic cellular functions.

Step 6: Storing Excess Glucose

But what happens if you consume more carbohydrates than your body needs at that moment? Your body has a clever way of storing this excess glucose for later use. First, glucose is stored in the liver and muscles as glycogen. Glycogen is like your body's backup energy reserve, ready to be tapped into when you need an extra boost of energy, such as during intense exercise or between meals.

If your glycogen stores are full and there's still excess glucose, your body converts this surplus into fat and stores it in adipose tissue. This is one reason why consuming too many carbs without burning them off through physical activity can lead to weight gain.

Glycogen plays a vital role in your body's energy management. During exercise, especially high-intensity workouts, your body relies heavily on glycogen stores for quick energy. This is why athletes often focus on "carb loading" before a big event—to maximize their glycogen stores and ensure they have enough energy to sustain their performance.

The Glycemic Index: A Handy Tool

The glycemic index (GI) is a useful tool for understanding how different carbs affect your blood sugar levels. The GI measures how quickly a carbohydrate-containing food raises your blood sugar levels on a scale of 0 to 100 (Link, 2023).

- **Low GI foods (55 or less):** Cause a slower, more gradual increase in blood sugar levels. Examples include most fruits, vegetables, and whole grains.
- **Medium GI foods (56-69):** Have a moderate impact on blood sugar levels. Examples include brown rice, sweet potatoes, and whole wheat bread.
- **High GI foods (70 or above):** Cause a rapid spike in blood sugar levels. Examples include white bread, sugary cereals, and instant rice.

Choosing low-to-medium-GI foods helps maintain steady energy levels and can prevent the rollercoaster of blood sugar spikes and crashes.

Carbs and Weight Management

Carbs often get a bad rap in weight management, but balance and choosing the right types are key. Understanding how your body processes and uses carbohydrates helps you make informed decisions that support your health and fitness goals. Carb cycling is an effective strategy, allowing you to enjoy the benefits of carbs without overconsumption. Carbohydrates are crucial for digestion, absorption, energy production, and storage, keeping your body fueled and functioning optimally. Selecting the right types of carbs and timing your intake strategically can enhance performance, support recovery, and manage weight effectively.

Choosing the Right Carbs: Complex vs. Simple

We've touched on the basics of simple and complex carbs, but now it's time to really dig into how to choose the right carbohydrates for your diet.

Complex carbs are made up of longer chains of sugar molecules (polysaccharides), which take longer for the body to break down and digest. Slower digestion provides a steadier release of glucose into the bloodstream, leading to more sustained energy levels. Complex carbs include:

> **Starch:** Found in foods like potatoes, corn, and grains.
> **Fiber:** Found in fruits, vegetables, legumes, and whole grains.

Complex carbohydrates are generally considered more beneficial for your health than simple carbs for several reasons:

Sustained energy levels: The steady release of glucose into the bloodstream helps maintain stable energy levels throughout the day, preventing the spikes and crashes associated with simple carbs.

Rich in nutrients: Complex carbs often come from whole, unprocessed foods that are rich in vitamins, minerals, and fiber. These nutrients are essential for overall health and can help reduce the risk of chronic diseases.

Better blood sugar control: The slower digestion of complex carbs helps prevent rapid spikes in blood sugar levels, making them a better choice for managing blood sugar levels and reducing the risk of type 2 diabetes.

Promotes digestive health: Foods high in complex carbs are often also high in fiber, which is important for maintaining a healthy digestive system. Fiber helps regulate bowel movements, prevent constipation, and support a healthy gut microbiome.

Let's look at some examples of complex carbs and how you can incorporate them into your diet:

> ***Whole Grains:*** Whole grains are an excellent source of complex carbs, fiber, and essential nutrients.
> • Quinoa: A complete protein that is also high in fiber and various vitamins and minerals
> • Brown rice: A great source of magnesium, phosphorus, and B vitamins
> • Oats: Rich in fiber and antioxidants, oats are perfect for breakfast or as a base for energy bars

Vegetables: Vegetables are not only rich in complex carbs but also packed with vitamins, minerals, and fiber
• Sweet potatoes: High in vitamins A and C, fiber, and antioxidants
• Broccoli: A cruciferous vegetable loaded with vitamins K and C, folate, and fiber
• Spinach: A leafy green rich in iron, calcium, and vitamins A and C

Legumes: Legumes are a fantastic source of plant-based protein, fiber, and complex carbs
• Lentils: High in protein, iron, and folate, lentils are great for soups and stews
• Chickpeas: Versatile and nutritious, chickpeas can be used in salads, hummus, and stews
• Black beans: Rich in protein, fiber, and antioxidants, black beans are perfect for soups and burritos

Simple carbs consist of one or two sugar molecules (monosaccharides and disaccharides) and are quickly broken down by the body, leading to quick spikes in blood sugar levels, followed by crashes, which is why they're often referred to as "quick energy" sources. Simple carbs include:

• **Glucose:** Found in fruits and vegetables
• **Fructose:** Found in fruits, honey, and root vegetables
• **Sucrose:** Common table sugar found in candies and processed foods
• **Lactose:** The sugar found in milk and dairy products

While simple carbs are not inherently bad, they are often consumed in excess due to their presence in processed and sugary foods. Here are some reasons to be cautious with simple carbs:

Rapid blood sugar spikes: Simple carbs are quickly digested, leading to rapid spikes in blood sugar levels. This can result in energy crashes, increased hunger, and cravings for more sugar.

Low nutritional value: Many foods high in simple carbs, such as candies, sugary cereals, and soft drinks, offer little nutritional value. They are often high in calories but low in essential nutrients, which can contribute to weight gain and poor health.

Increased risk of chronic diseases: A diet high in simple carbs and added sugars has been linked to an increased risk of chronic diseases such as obesity, type 2 diabetes, and heart disease.

Here are some common examples of simple carbs and how to consume them mindfully:

Fruit: Fruits contain natural sugars but also provide fiber, vitamins, and antioxidants. Enjoy them in moderation.
• Berries: Blueberries, strawberries, and raspberries are lower in sugar compared to other fruits and high in fiber.
• Apples: A great source of fiber and vitamin C.
• Bananas: Rich in potassium and a good source of quick energy.

Dairy: Milk and dairy products contain lactose, a natural sugar. They also provide calcium, protein, and other essential nutrients.
• Greek yogurt: High in protein and can be enjoyed with fruits and nuts for added fiber.
• Milk: A good source of calcium and vitamin D but opt for unsweetened versions to avoid added sugars.

Processed & Sugary Foods: These should be limited as much as possible due to their high sugar content and low nutritional value.
• Candy: Provides quick energy but can lead to a sugar crash.
• Sugary cereals: Often high in added sugars and low in fiber.
• Soft drinks: High in added sugars and calories with no nutritional benefits.

Balancing Complex and Simple Carbs in Your Diet

Although it's important to prioritize complex carbs for their nutritional benefits, simple carbs can also have a place in a balanced diet. Here's how to incorporate both types of carbs wisely:

Focus on whole foods: Make whole, unprocessed foods the foundation of your diet. These foods are typically rich in complex carbs, fiber, vitamins, and minerals.

Use simple carbs strategically: Simple carbs can be beneficial during workouts for quick energy. For example, having a banana before a workout can provide a quick energy boost without causing a sugar crash.

Read labels: Be mindful of added sugars in processed foods by reading nutrition labels. Aim to choose products with minimal added sugars and more natural ingredients.

Balance your meals: Pair simple carbs with protein and healthy fats to slow down digestion and maintain stable blood sugar levels. For example, enjoy a piece of fruit with a handful of nuts or some Greek yogurt.

Here are some tips to help you make the best carb choices for your health and fitness goals:

• **Plan your meals:** Planning your meals in advance can help ensure you're getting a balanced intake of complex carbs, protein, and healthy fats. Include a variety of whole grains, vegetables, and legumes in your meal prep.

• **Snack smart:** Keep healthy snacks on hand, like cut-up veggies, fruits, and nuts. This makes it easier to reach for nutrient-dense options when hunger strikes.

• **Cook at home:** Preparing meals at home gives you control over the ingredients and allows you to focus on whole, unprocessed foods. Experiment with new recipes that incorporate complex carbs.

• **Listen to your body:** Pay attention to how different carbs make you feel. If you notice energy crashes after consuming simple carbs, try switching to more complex carbs for sustained energy.

Choosing the right carbohydrates is key to supporting your health and fitness goals. By focusing on whole, unprocessed foods and balancing your carb intake with protein and healthy fats, you can create a well-rounded diet that supports your body's needs. Remember, the goal is to find a balance that works for you and helps you feel your best.

Now, let's take things a step further. Diet alone can only get you so far; to truly maximize your results, you need to pair your nutritional plan with the right workouts. In the next chapter, we'll explore essential workouts that complement your carb-cycling diet including exercise routines that can help you build muscle, burn fat, and boost your metabolism.

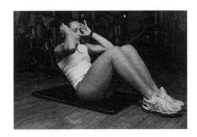

Chapter Four

Essential Workouts to Complement Your Diet

Exercise will take your carb cycling plan from good to absolutely transformative! Exercise and diet go hand in hand, and when paired correctly, they create a synergy that propels you toward your health and fitness goals.

Let's explore different types of workouts, best practices for scheduling them, and ensure you have a comprehensive understanding of how to seamlessly integrate exercise into your carb cycling plan.

How Exercise Enhances the Effects of Carb Cycling

Exercise is essential for maintaining health and it can power boost your carb cycling efforts to help you see those physical results faster. If you're serious about your weight loss journey, combining a structured exercise routine with your carb cycling plan is the key you've been looking for. Carb cycling and exercise are like two peas in a pod—they work together beautifully to enhance each other's effects. Here's why:

Maximizes Energy and Performance: On high-carb days, you fuel your body with carbohydrates, your primary energy source. This is ideal for high-intensity workouts like weightlifting or interval training, as the consumed carbs convert to glycogen, stored in your muscles and liver.

This allows you to push harder and longer during exercise, maximizing performance, muscle growth, and fat loss.

Enhances Fat Burning: Low-carb days tap into your body's fat stores for energy. Reduced carb intake lowers insulin levels, prompting fat burning. This is perfect for cardio or steady-state exercise, accelerating fat loss. Alternating between high- and low-carb days while aligning your workouts accordingly trains your body to efficiently burn both glycogen and fat, which is essential for achieving and maintaining weight-loss goals.

Boosts Metabolism: Exercise, especially strength training, significantly impacts your metabolism by building lean muscle mass, increasing your resting metabolic rate (RMR). This means you burn more calories at rest. Combining this with carb cycling keeps your metabolism high. High-carb days support intense training and muscle growth, while low-carb days enhance fat burning and metabolic efficiency.

Prevents Plateaus: Weight-loss plateaus can stall progress, but carb cycling, and varied workouts help prevent this. Changing your carb intake and varying exercises keeps your body guessing, preventing your metabolism from adapting to a single routine and stalling.

The Psychological Benefits of Exercise

In addition to the physical benefits, exercise also has a profound impact on your mental well-being. Here's how:

Reduces stress and anxiety: Exercise releases endorphins, often referred to as the "feel-good" hormones. These endorphins help reduce stress and anxiety, making you feel happier and more relaxed. This is particularly important during a weight loss journey, which can sometimes feel challenging and stressful (Washington, 2022).

Boosts confidence: As you progress in your fitness journey and start seeing physical results, your confidence will naturally increase. This boost in self-esteem can motivate you to stay consistent with your carb cycling and exercise plan (Mayo Clinic Staff, 2021).

Enhances focus and productivity: Regular exercise has been shown to improve cognitive function, memory, and overall brain health. This means you'll be more focused and productive in your daily activities, helping you stay on track with your goals (Mandolesi et al., 2018).

Here are some practical tips to help you make the most of your exercise routine and carb cycling plan:

• **Plan your workouts:** Schedule your workouts in advance, aligning them with your high-carb and low-carb days. This helps ensure you're maximizing the benefits of both your diet and exercise routine.

• **Listen to your body:** Pay attention to how your body feels and adjust your workouts accordingly. If you're feeling particularly fatigued on a low-carb day, opt for a lighter workout or an active rest day.

• **Stay consistent:** Consistency is key. Stick to your plan, but also be flexible and make adjustments as needed. Progress takes time, so be patient with yourself and stay committed.

• **Mix it up:** Variety keeps things interesting and prevents your body from adapting to a single routine. Incorporate different types of workouts to keep your muscles challenged and your mind engaged.

Combining exercise with carb cycling creates a powerful synergy that enhances both fat loss and muscle gain. Aligning your workouts with your carb intake maximizes energy levels, boosts metabolism, and accelerates progress.

Workout Routines

High-Carb Days: High-Intensity Interval Training (HIIT)

High-carb days are perfect for those powerhouse sessions that push your limits and maximize your performance. One of the best types of workouts to incorporate these days is high-intensity interval training, or HIIT. Let's dive into what HIIT is, the incredible benefits it offers, and some specific workouts you can try.

What is HIIT?

HIIT, or High-Intensity Interval Training, alternates short bursts of intense activity with brief rest periods. This workout keeps your heart rate up and burns more fat in less time. During the high-intensity intervals, you exert maximum effort, and then rest briefly. For example, sprint for 30 seconds, walk for 60 seconds, and repeat. The goal is to push your limits during intense phases, creating an efficient workout that boosts metabolism and enhances fitness.

Benefits of HIIT Exercising

HIIT offers a range of benefits that make it a standout choice for high-carb days. Here's why you should consider incorporating HIIT into your routine (Tinsley, 2017):

Burn a significant number of calories in a short period of time: One of the biggest advantages of HIIT is its efficiency. You can burn a lot of calories in a relatively short amount of time. Studies have shown that a 30-minute HIIT session can burn more calories than longer, moderate-intensity cardio workouts. This makes it an excellent option for those who are short on time but still want to get a great workout in.

Long-lasting elevated metabolic rate: HIIT not only burns a lot of calories during the workout but also keeps your metabolic rate elevated for hours afterward. This phenomenon, known as excess post-exercise oxygen consumption (EPOC), means your body continues to burn calories at an increased rate even after you've finished exercising. It's like getting a bonus calorie burn!

Lose fat: HIIT is highly effective at burning fat. A combination of intense effort and an increased metabolic rate helps your body tap into its fat stores for energy. Research has shown that HIIT can help reduce both subcutaneous fat (the fat under your skin) and visceral fat (the dangerous fat around your organs).

Gain muscle: While HIIT is primarily known for its fat-burning capabilities, it also helps in building lean muscle mass, especially when it includes strength-based movements like squats, lunges, and kettlebell swings. Maintaining or increasing muscle mass is crucial for boosting your metabolism and achieving a toned physique.

Improve oxygen intake: HIIT enhances your body's ability to use oxygen. By pushing your cardiovascular system during intense intervals, you improve your VO_2 max (the maximum amount of oxygen your body can utilize during exercise). This leads to better endurance and overall fitness.

Lower heart rate and blood pressure: Regular HIIT workouts can lead to significant improvements in heart health. Studies have shown that HIIT can help lower resting heart rate and reduce blood pressure, contributing to a healthier cardiovascular system.

Enhance aerobic and anaerobic performance: HIIT boosts both aerobic (endurance) and anaerobic (high-intensity, short-duration) performance. By challenging both energy systems, you become more versatile and better prepared for various physical activities.

Now that you understand the benefits of HIIT, let's look at some specific exercises you can include in your HIIT routine. The great thing about HIIT is its flexibility—you can mix and match different exercises to keep your workouts interesting and challenging.

Lunges

How to do it: Stand with your feet hip-width apart. Step forward with one leg and lower your body until both knees are bent at a 90-degree angle. Push through the heel of your front foot to return to the starting position, then switch legs.

HIIT variation: Perform lunges for 30 seconds, then rest for 30 seconds. Repeat for 4–5 rounds.

Mountain Climbers

How to do it: Start in a plank position with your hands under your shoulders and your body in a straight line. Quickly drive one knee toward your chest, then switch legs as if you're "climbing" in place.

HIIT variation: Perform mountain climbers for 30 seconds, then rest for 30 seconds. Repeat for 4–5 rounds.

Squats

How to do it: Stand with your feet shoulder-width apart. Lower your body by bending your knees and pushing your hips back, as if sitting in a chair. Keep your chest up and your knees over your toes. Return to the starting position.

HIIT variation: Perform squats for 30 seconds, then rest for 30 seconds. Repeat for 4–5 rounds.

Jumping rope

How to do it: Hold the handles of the rope with your hands at your sides and the rope behind you. Swing the rope over your head and jump as it passes under your feet. Keep a steady rhythm and maintain a light bounce.

HIIT variation: Jump rope for 30 seconds, then rest for 30 seconds. Repeat for 4–5 rounds.

Jumping Jacks

How to do it: Stand with your feet together and your hands at your sides. Jump and spread your legs while raising your arms overhead. Jump again to return to the starting position.

HIIT variation: Perform jumping jacks for 30 seconds, then rest for 30 seconds. Repeat for 4–5 rounds.

Kettlebell Swing

How to do it: Stand with your feet shoulder-width apart and hold a kettlebell with both hands in front of you. Bend your knees slightly and hinge at your hips to swing the kettlebell back between your legs. Then, thrust your hips forward to swing the kettlebell up to shoulder height.

HIIT variation: Perform kettlebell swings for 30 seconds, then rest for 30 seconds. Repeat for 4–5 rounds.

Russian Twists

How to do it: Sit on the floor with your knees bent and your feet flat. Lean back slightly and hold a weight, exercise band or medicine ball with both hands. Twist your torso to the right, then to the left, tapping the weight on the floor beside you each time.

HIIT variation: Perform Russian twists for 30 seconds, then rest for 30 seconds. Repeat for 4–5 rounds.

Burpees

How to do it: Start standing, then drop into a squat position with your hands on the floor. Kick your feet back into a plank position, perform a push-up, then jump your feet back to your hands and explosively jump up into the air.

HIIT variation: Perform burpees for 30 seconds, then rest for 30 seconds. Repeat for 4–5 rounds.

Creating a HIIT Workout Routine

Here's how you can structure a HIIT workout using the exercises above:

Warm Up (5-10 Minutes)

1. Jumping jacks

2. Arm circles

3. Leg swings

4. High knees

5. Dynamic stretches (e.g., lunges with a twist)

HIIT Session (20-30 Minutes):

Perform each exercise for 30 seconds, followed by 30 seconds of rest. Complete the circuit 4-5 times.

1. Lunges

2. Mountain climbers

3. Squats

4. Jumping rope

5. Jumping jacks

6. Kettlebell swing

7. Russian twists

8. Burpees

Cool Down (5-10 Minutes)

1. Light jogging or walking

2. Static stretching (e.g., hamstring stretch, quadriceps stretch, shoulder stretch)

3. Deep breathing exercises

High-carb days are ideal for harnessing the power of HIIT. Incorporating high-intensity interval training into your routine maximizes calorie burn, boosts metabolism, and enhances both aerobic and anaerobic fitness. The variety and intensity of HIIT make it an effective and exciting addition to your carb cycling plan.

Low-Carb Days: Low-Intensity Steady State Cardio (LISS)

Let's talk about how you can make the most of your low-carb days with low-intensity steady state (LISS) cardio. LISS cardio is an excellent complement to your carb cycling plan, particularly on low-carb days when you're focusing on fat burning and recovery.

What Is Low-Intensity Steady-State Cardio?

Low-Intensity Steady State (LISS) cardio is a form of cardiovascular exercise performed at a low to moderate intensity for a continuous, extended period. Unlike high-intensity interval training (HIIT), which involves short bursts of intense activity followed by rest, LISS cardio keeps your heart rate relatively steady, typically around 50 to 65 percent of your maximum heart rate (Lindberg, 2019).

This type of training is not new—it's been around for decades under various names, such as steady-state training (SST), continuous cardiovascular exercise, or long slow distance (LSD) training. It's the opposite of HIIT in terms of intensity and structure, making it a perfect fit for those days when you're not consuming as many carbs and need a gentler, yet effective, workout.

Benefits of Low-Intensity Steady State Cardio

LISS cardio comes with a plethora of benefits, making it an excellent addition to your fitness regimen, especially on low-carb days. Here are some key advantages (Lindberg, 2019):

Improves cardiovascular health: LISS cardio helps strengthen your heart and improve blood circulation. Regularly engaging in this type of exercise can lower your risk of cardiovascular diseases by improving your heart's efficiency and reducing blood pressure. It's a heart-healthy way to stay active without the intensity of high-impact workouts.

Burns fat: One of the primary benefits of LISS cardio is its effectiveness in burning fat. During low-intensity exercise, your body primarily uses fat as fuel rather than glycogen stored in your muscles. LISS is an excellent choice for low-carb days when glycogen stores are lower. Engaging in steady-state cardio helps you tap into your fat reserves, promoting weight loss and improved body composition.

Builds endurance: LISS cardio helps build endurance by training your aerobic system over longer periods of time. This is particularly beneficial if you're preparing for endurance events like marathons, triathlons, or long-distance cycling. Regularly incorporating LISS into your routine improves your stamina and helps you perform better in long-duration activities.

Reduces stress: Exercise, in general, is a fantastic stress reliever, and LISS cardio is no exception. The steady, rhythmic nature of LISS can have a calming effect, reducing levels of stress hormones like cortisol. Whether it's a long walk in the park, a gentle swim, or a leisurely bike ride, LISS cardio provides a mental break and promotes relaxation.

Accessible for all fitness levels: One of the most appealing aspects of LISS cardio is its accessibility. It's suitable for people of all fitness levels and physical limitations. Whether you're a beginner, recovering from an injury, or just prefer a gentler workout, LISS allows you to stay active without overexerting yourself. It's a low-barrier way to incorporate cardiovascular exercise into your routine.

Joint friendly: Because LISS cardio involves low-impact activities, it's easier on your joints compared to high-impact exercises like running or jumping. This makes it a great option for those with joint issues or those looking to avoid high-impact strain. Activities like walking, cycling, and swimming can all provide an excellent cardiovascular workout while being gentle on the body.

There are many ways to incorporate LISS cardio into your fitness routine. Here are some examples of activities you can try:

Walking is one of the simplest and most accessible forms of LISS cardio. Whether it's a brisk walk around your neighborhood, a hike in the hills, or a stroll on the treadmill, walking can be done almost anywhere and requires no special equipment. Aim for 45 to 60 minutes at a moderate pace to reap the benefits.

Cycling, whether on a stationary bike or out on the road, is a great low-impact cardio exercise. Set a steady pace and enjoy a scenic ride or a focused session at the gym. This activity is excellent for building leg strength and endurance while being gentle on the joints.

Swimming is another excellent form of LISS cardio. The resistance of the water provides a full-body workout without putting stress on your joints. Swim laps at a steady pace for an extended period, focusing on smooth, controlled movements.

Using an **elliptical trainer** is a great way to get a low-impact cardio workout. It mimics the motion of running without the impact, making it a joint-friendly option. Set a moderate resistance level and maintain a steady pace for 45 to 60 minutes.

Rowing is a fantastic full-body workout that can be performed at low intensity. Whether you use a rowing machine or row on water, aim for a continuous, steady pace to improve cardiovascular health and endurance.

Hiking on trails with gentle inclines provides an excellent way to engage in LISS cardio while enjoying the great outdoors. It's a great way to combine exercise with nature, and the varied terrain can add a bit of challenge while keeping the intensity low.

How to Incorporate LISS Cardio into Your Routine

Incorporating LISS cardio into your fitness plan is straightforward and easily adaptable to work with your schedule. Here's how you can get started:

Schedule regular sessions: If you're a beginner, aim for three LISS cardio sessions per week. As you progress, you can adjust the frequency and duration based on your fitness level and goals. For intermediate to advanced levels, including one or two sessions of LISS cardio along with your HIIT or strength training sessions can provide a balanced approach.

Combine with strength training: While LISS cardio is excellent for improving cardiovascular health and burning fat, it's also important to include strength training exercises in your routine. Aim to engage in strength training for all major muscle groups at least 2-3 days per week. This combination helps build muscle, boost metabolism, and improve overall fitness.

Use cardio equipment: If you belong to a gym or have home cardio equipment like a treadmill, elliptical, rower, or exercise bike, you can easily incorporate LISS cardio. Set the machine to a moderate pace and maintain it for 45 to 60 minutes. This allows for a convenient and controlled workout environment.

Outdoor activities: Prefer the great outdoors? Hit the pavement for a long run, bike ride, or walk. Hiking and swimming are also excellent outdoor LISS options. The key is to maintain a steady pace for an extended period to maximize the benefits.

Mix it up: To prevent boredom and keep things interesting, vary your LISS activities. Rotate between different exercises like walking, cycling, and swimming. This variety keeps your workouts engaging and challenges your body in different ways.

Here are some tips to help you get the most out of your LISS cardio sessions:

• **Monitor your heart rate:** To ensure you're staying within the low-intensity range, monitor your heart rate. Aim for 50 to 65 percent of your maximum heart rate. This can be calculated as 220 minus your age, then multiplied by the desired percentage. Using a heart rate monitor can help you stay on track.

- **Stay consistent:** Consistency is key to seeing results. Make LISS cardio a regular part of your routine and stick to your schedule. Over time, you'll notice improvements in your endurance, cardiovascular health, and overall fitness.

- **Listen to your body:** Pay attention to how your body feels during and after your workouts. If you experience any pain or discomfort, adjust the intensity or duration of your exercise. LISS should be challenging yet comfortable enough to be performed regularly.

- **Hydrate and fuel:** Even though LISS cardio is lower intensity, it's still important to stay hydrated and fuel your body properly. Drink plenty of water before, during, and after your workouts, and consume a balanced diet to support your energy needs.

- **Enjoy the process:** LISS cardio can be a relaxing and enjoyable form of exercise. Use this time to unwind, listen to your favorite music or podcast, or enjoy the scenery if you're exercising outdoors. Finding joy in your workouts makes it easier to stay committed.

Adding LISS cardio to your routine is easy and can be customized to fit your schedule and preferences. Activities like walking, cycling, swimming, or using cardio equipment work well, as long as you maintain a steady pace for an extended time. This method improves overall fitness and supports both weight loss and health goals.

I know that starting and sticking to a new fitness regimen can feel overwhelming. Well, you're not alone in this. Many of us face the same challenges—finding the time, staying motivated, and figuring out the best way to see results without feeling burnt out. Remember, every step you take, no matter how small, is a step toward your goals. You're here, learning and taking proactive steps to improve your health, and that's something to be incredibly proud of.

There are many common hurdles we all face. Maybe you're juggling a busy work schedule, family responsibilities, or social commitments, and finding time to work out feels like an impossible task. Or perhaps you're struggling with motivation, questioning whether all this effort will really pay off. It's natural to have these doubts and challenges, but like I said before, integrating exercise with your carb cycling plan isn't about being perfect; it's about finding a balance that works for you.

On high-carb days, you have the perfect opportunity to push yourself with HIIT workouts. These intense sessions don't need to take hours of your day. Even just 20–30 minutes of dedicated effort can leave you feeling invigorated and accomplished. Plus, the metabolic boost you get from HIIT can keep you burning calories long after you've finished your workout.

Then there are the low-carb days, where the focus shifts to steady, gentle movements that still provide tremendous benefits. LISS cardio can feel like a breath of fresh air. It's a chance to clear your mind with a long walk, a swim, or a bike ride. It's not just about burning calories; it's about taking care of your mental health and giving your body a break while still staying active.

It's okay to have days where you don't hit every workout perfectly or days where you need a little extra rest. What's important is that you're creating a routine that fits into your life and makes you feel good. It's about building habits that are sustainable and enjoyable, rather than forcing yourself into a rigid schedule that feels like a chore.

You've got the knowledge and the tools now. Take it one day at a time, listen to your body, and celebrate your progress along the way.

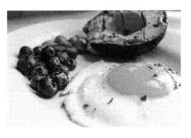

Chapter Five

Customizing Your Diet to Fit Your Lifestyle

You know what's even more powerful than a perfectly structured diet? A diet that fits seamlessly into your life adapts to your needs and supports your goals in a way that feels natural and sustainable.

The fact is —no two people are the same. We all have different goals, preferences, and challenges when it comes to diet and exercise. That's why a one-size-fits-all approach rarely works in the long run. To truly succeed, you need a plan that's as dynamic and adaptable as you are.

This chapter explores creating a personalized carb cycling plan tailored to your unique goals, whether for weight loss, muscle gain, or athletic performance. We'll also address special dietary needs like vegetarianism, allergies, and sustainability, ensuring your plan is effective and enjoyable for the long term.

Carb Cycling for Different Goals

Carb cycling isn't just a one-trick pony—it's a versatile tool that can help you achieve a variety of fitness goals, including losing weight, gaining muscle, or enhancing athletic performance. Let's break down how carb cycling can be tailored to support each of these objectives, ensuring you get the most out of your diet and training efforts.

Weight Loss: If shedding those extra pounds is your primary goal, carb cycling can be incredibly effective. One of the key benefits of carb cycling for weight loss is its ability to improve fat burning while maintaining muscle mass.

When following a low-carb diet, your body uses fat as its primary fuel source, a process called ketosis that enhances fat burning. On low-carb days, depleted glycogen stores prompt your body to burn more fat for energy. This approach is particularly useful for breaking through weight-loss plateaus caused by metabolic adaptation to a consistent calorie deficit.

However, the trick with carb cycling is to periodically reintroduce high-carb days. According to a 2019 study published in *Sports*, when you're in a calorie-deficit state for an extended period, your body's hormones—particularly leptin—signal your brain to minimize weight loss by burning fewer calories (Peos et al., 2019). This process, known as adaptive thermogenesis, can make sustained weight loss challenging. Incorporating high-carb days temporarily increases blood leptin levels, potentially boosting metabolism and preventing the body from entering a metabolic slowdown.

While more research is needed to fully understand the relationship between carb cycling and leptin levels, the current evidence suggests that strategically timed high-carb days can help maintain a healthy metabolic rate and improve the body's ability to burn fat as fuel.

Muscle Gain: For those looking to build muscle, carb cycling offers a strategic approach to optimizing your nutrition and training efforts. Gaining muscle requires not just protein but also a sufficient amount of carbohydrates to fuel intense workouts and support recovery.

A 2017 study highlighted in *Medical News Today* suggests that competitive bodybuilders who utilize carbohydrate refeeds (periods of increased carb intake) believe it enhances fat loss and boosts training performance (Mitchell et al., 2017). High-carb days replenish glycogen stores providing the energy needed for intense strength training, enabling you to lift heavier and train harder while aiding in muscle recovery and growth.

During these high-carb periods, insulin plays a crucial role in muscle protein synthesis. Insulin helps transport amino acids into muscle cells, promoting muscle repair and growth post-workout. This is why consuming carbs after a workout, along with protein, is essential for optimal muscle recovery.

Maintaining adequate protein intake during low-carb consumption days ensures muscle tissue is preserved. Balancing high and low-carb days supports muscle gain without excess fat accumulation, resulting in a leaner, more defined physique.

Athletic Performance and Endurance: For athletes and those looking to enhance their athletic performance, carb cycling can provide the necessary fuel for high-intensity workouts and endurance events while also promoting efficient fat utilization.

Athletes often face a dilemma: they need carbohydrates for peak performance, especially during high-intensity, short-duration exercises, but they also want the benefits of a low-carb diet for enhanced fat burning and aerobic adaptation. Carb cycling offers a solution by allowing athletes to strategically consume carbs to fuel their most demanding training sessions and competitions.

According to experts, training in a low-carb state can boost fat-burning capacity and accelerate aerobic adaptation (Martins, 2019). However, for high-intensity workouts, having sufficient glycogen stores is crucial. Consuming carbs before such workouts ensures that your body has the necessary fuel to perform at its best. Interestingly, research indicates that even the presence of carbs in the mouth can enhance performance by activating brain regions involved in reward and motor control (Martins, 2019).

Post-exercise carbohydrate consumption aids in glycogen resynthesis and protein synthesis, facilitating faster recovery. This is vital for athletes who need to perform consistently at high levels. Incorporating high-carb days ensures that athletes' intense training sessions are of high quality, enhancing overall performance and recovery.

Tailoring Carb Cycling to Your Goals

Now that we've explored how carb cycling can support weight loss, muscle gain, and athletic performance, let's talk about how you can tailor this approach to your specific goals.

Weight Loss

• **High-carb days:** Plan these days around your most intense workouts. Increase your carb intake to 200–300 grams per day, focusing on complex carbs like sweet potatoes, brown rice, and whole grains. This helps replenish glycogen stores and boost metabolism.

• **Low-carb days:** Focus on consuming lean proteins, healthy fats, and plenty of non-starchy vegetables. Aim for a carb intake that keeps your body in a fat-burning mode, typically around 50–100 grams of carbs per day.

• **Calorie management:** Ensure you're in a calorie deficit overall, even with the high-carb days. Monitor your portion sizes and choose nutrient-dense foods to keep you full and satisfied.

Muscle Gain

• **High-carb days:** Align these days with your heavy lifting or most intense training sessions. Aim for a higher carb intake, around 300–400 grams per day, to fuel your workouts and promote muscle protein synthesis.

• **Low-carb days:** Keep your carb intake moderate, around 100–150 grams per day, focusing on maintaining protein intake to support muscle repair. Include healthy fats to meet your calorie needs without adding excessive carbs.

• **Protein intake:** Ensure you're consuming enough protein each day, ideally 1.2–2.2 grams per kilogram of body weight, to support muscle growth and recovery.

Athletic Performance

• **Training phase:** During your training phase, use low-carb days to enhance fat-burning capacity and aerobic adaptation. Keep your carb intake moderate to low, around 100–150 grams per day.

• **Competition phase:** Before competitions or high-intensity training sessions, switch to high-carb days. Increase your carb intake to 300–400 grams per day to ensure your glycogen stores are fully replenished.

• **Recovery:** Post-competition or intense workouts, focus on balanced meals with both carbs and protein to aid recovery and glycogen re-synthesis. This ensures you're ready for your next training session.

Carb Cycling for Special Diets

One of the most empowering aspects of carb cycling is its flexibility—it can be tailored to fit virtually any dietary need or preference. Whether you're vegetarian, vegan, gluten-free, or have other specific dietary restrictions, carb cycling can be adapted to ensure you still achieve your health and fitness goals.

Vegan & Vegetarian Adaptations

If you follow a vegan or vegetarian diet, you might wonder how you can successfully incorporate carb cycling without compromising your dietary choices. The good news is that it's entirely possible, and you can still enjoy a variety of nutrient-dense foods while cycling your carbs.

One of the main concerns with a plant-based diet is getting enough protein. Fortunately, there are plenty of high-protein plant foods that can fit perfectly into your carb cycling plan. Here are some excellent sources:

• Legumes: Beans, lentils, and chickpeas are all high in protein and fiber. They can be used in soups, salads, and as a base for veggie burgers.

• Tofu and tempeh: These soy-based products are versatile and protein-packed. Use them in stir-fries, sandwiches, or as a meat substitute in various dishes.

• Nuts and seeds: Almonds, chia seeds, flaxseeds, and hemp seeds provide protein, healthy fats, and fiber. They can be added to smoothies, oatmeal, and salads.

• Quinoa: This grain is a complete protein, meaning it contains all nine essential amino acids. It's perfect for salads, bowls, or as a side dish.

Here's an example of how you might structure your meals on high-carb and low-carb days as a vegetarian or vegan:

High-Carb

Breakfast
Overnight oats made with almond milk, chia seeds, and topped with fresh berries and a drizzle of maple syrup

Snack
A smoothie with spinach, banana, plant-based protein powder, and a handful of nuts

Lunch
Quinoa and black bean salad with mixed greens, cherry tomatoes, avocado, and a lime vinaigrette

Snack
Apple slices with almond butter

Dinner
Chickpea and vegetable stir-fry served over brown rice

Low-Carb

> **Breakfast**
> Scrambled tofu with spinach, mushrooms, and tomatoes, served with a side of avocado
> **Snack**
> Celery sticks with hummus
> **Lunch**
> Mixed green salad with roasted vegetables, quinoa, and a tahini dressing
> **Snack**
> A handful of mixed nuts
> **Dinner**
> Lentil and vegetable curry served over cauliflower rice

Gluten-Free Adaptations

For those with celiac disease or gluten sensitivity, maintaining a gluten-free diet is essential. Carb cycling can be easily adapted to fit a gluten-free lifestyle by focusing on naturally gluten-free carbs and snacks.

There are many delicious and nutritious gluten-free carbohydrate sources to choose from. Here are some options:

• Quinoa: A versatile and complete protein that can be used in salads, as a side dish, or even in breakfast bowls.
• Sweet potatoes: High in fiber and vitamins, they can be baked, roasted, or mashed.
• Brown rice: A staple gluten-free grain that pairs well with a variety of dishes.
• Oats: Make sure to choose gluten-free oats for your breakfasts and snacks.
• Fruits and vegetables: Naturally gluten-free and packed with essential nutrients and fiber.
• Legumes: Beans, lentils, and chickpeas are all great sources of carbs and protein.

Here's how you can structure your meals on high-carb and low-carb days while keeping them gluten-free:

High-Carb

> **Breakfast**
> Gluten-free oats topped with fresh fruit, chia seeds, and a drizzle of honey
> **Snack**
> A smoothie with gluten-free protein powder, spinach, banana, and a splash of almond milk
> **Lunch**
> Quinoa salad with mixed greens, cherry tomatoes, cucumber, and a lemon vinaigrette
> **Snack**
> Rice cakes with almond butter and sliced bananas
> **Dinner**
> Grilled chicken with sweet potato fries and a side of steamed broccoli

Low-Carb

> **Breakfast**
> Greek yogurt with chia seeds, nuts, and a few berries
> **Snack**
> Carrot sticks with hummus
> **Lunch**
> Spinach salad with grilled salmon, avocado, and a balsamic vinaigrette
> **Snack**
> A handful of mixed nuts
> **Dinner**
> Zucchini noodles with turkey meatballs and marinara sauce

Dairy-Free:

If you're lactose intolerant or follow a dairy-free diet, you can easily adapt to carb cycling by choosing plant-based alternatives.

Breakfast
Smoothie with almond milk, dairy-free protein powder, spinach, and a banana
Snack
Apple slices with almond butter
Lunch
Chickpea salad with mixed greens, cherry tomatoes, cucumber, and a lemon-tahini dressing
Snack
Hummus with carrot sticks
Dinner
Stir-fried tofu with broccoli, bell peppers, and brown rice

Nut-Free:

For those with nut allergies, focus on seeds and other protein sources

---

Breakfast
Greek yogurt with sunflower seeds, fresh fruit, and honey
Snack
Celery sticks with seed butter (like sunflower seed butter)
Lunch
Quinoa salad with mixed greens, chickpeas, cucumber, and a lemon vinaigrette
Snack
Rice cakes with seed butter and sliced strawberries
Dinner
Grilled chicken with roasted sweet potatoes and steamed green beans

---

Keto Adaptations

If you're following a ketogenic diet, you can still incorporate carb cycling by having low-carb days that align with your keto goals and slightly higher-carb days to replenish glycogen stores:

Moderate-Carb

Breakfast
Greek yogurt with a handful of berries and chia seeds
Snack
A small apple with cheese slices
Lunch
Quinoa and black bean salad with mixed greens and a lime vinaigrette
Snack
Rice cakes with almond butter
Dinner
Grilled chicken with a side of sweet potato fries and steamed broccoli

Low-Carb

Breakfast
Scrambled eggs with spinach and avocado
Snack
Cheese slices with cucumber
Lunch
Grilled chicken salad with mixed greens, avocado, and an olive oil vinaigrette
Snack
Olives and celery sticks
Dinner
Salmon with roasted asparagus and cauliflower mash

Carb cycling is a flexible and adaptable approach to nutrition that can fit a wide range of dietary needs and preferences. You can customize your carb cycling plan to support your health and fitness goals, regardless of being vegetarian, vegan, gluten-free, dairy-free, nut-free, or following a ketogenic diet.

Getting used to dietary changes can be challenging, but you've taken a significant step by exploring carb cycling and its potential to fit into your unique lifestyle. The key to making carb cycling work for you lies in flexibility and personalization. By allowing room for variety in your meal plans, finding healthy alternatives for your favorite foods, and making gradual adjustments, you can create a diet that's both effective and enjoyable. It's about finding a balance that fits into your life seamlessly without feeling restrictive or monotonous.

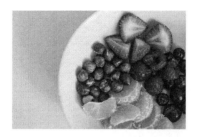

Chapter Six

Navigating Obstacles for Long-Term Success & Staying Committed

It's important that we take a minute to understand carb cycling is a way of life and let's be real—any significant lifestyle change comes with its fair share of challenges, and carb cycling is no exception. With the right strategies and mindset, you can overcome these obstacles and stay on track for the long haul. We're going to discuss how to maintain sustainability, navigate social situations, stay motivated and dive into practical solutions for managing hunger and cravings.

Carb cycling can be highly rewarding and a key component of your lifestyle, supporting your long-term health and fitness goals. However, without ensuring its sustainability, success will likely remain out of reach. Implementing the shared strategies in this chapter will prime you for achieving your goals and seeing success.

Social situations are a common challenge for all, from family gatherings to nights out with friends, it can be tough to stick to your carb cycling plan when everyone around you is indulging in tempting foods. I'll share some of my best tips for handling these scenarios gracefully so you can enjoy social events without feeling deprived or guilty. It's all about preparation, flexibility, and making smart choices that align with your goals.

Staying motivated is key to long-term success, and that means setting realistic, achievable goals and building a solid support system. We'll discuss how to set milestones that keep you motivated and celebrate your progress along the way. Plus, I'll show you how to build a network of support, whether it's friends, family, or online communities, to keep you encouraged and accountable.

Life isn't always predictable, and there will be times when things don't go according to plan. But with the strategies we'll cover in this chapter, you'll be equipped to handle setbacks and keep moving forward.

Hunger and cravings can be the biggest hurdles to maintaining any diet. We've all been there—those moments when a sudden craving hits, or your stomach starts growling at an inconvenient time. We'll explore strategies to manage these urges without derailing your progress. Whether it's learning how to structure your meals to keep you fuller for longer or finding healthy snacks that satisfy your cravings, you'll discover practical tips to keep hunger at bay.

As with any diet, there can be both mental and physical challenges and hurdles that may set you back. It's crucial to stay on course and remember *why* you're taking on this carb cycling journey. It's all about achieving your goals! Keeping your motivations and end goals in sight will help you push through tough times and stay committed.

Making Carb Cycling Sustainable

Creating sustainable dietary habits can be a challenge, but it's entirely possible with the right approach and mindset. Making carb cycling a lasting part of your lifestyle means crafting a meal and exercise plan that you can stick to long-term, without feeling deprived or overwhelmed.

Allow Flexibility in Your Meal Plans

Sticking to a rigid meal plan can lead to burnout and make it difficult to maintain your new dietary habits. Flexibility will keep things interesting and prevent monotony. Here's how you can incorporate flexibility into your meal plans:

Plan Variety and Choice: When planning your meals for the week, ensure you have a variety of foods and recipes to choose from. Instead of eating the same meals every day, rotate different dishes and experiment with new recipes. This keeps your meals exciting and prevents you from getting bored.

For example, on high-carb days, you might enjoy quinoa salad one day, sweet potato fries the next, and a hearty vegetable soup another day. On low-carb days, mix it up with different protein sources like grilled chicken, tofu stir-fry, and fish with steamed vegetables.

Build a Recipe Collection: Having a go-to collection of recipes can make meal planning easier and more enjoyable. Collect recipes that fit into both your high-carb and low-carb days, ensuring they're easy to prepare and delicious. With this approach, you'll always have a variety of meals to choose from without having to think too hard about what to cook.

Plan for Flexibility: Sometimes life happens, and you might not be able to stick to your planned meals. That's okay! Allow for flexibility by having some easy-to-make or ready-made meals on hand. This could be as simple as keeping frozen vegetables, pre-cooked grains, and canned beans in your pantry for quick meal options.

Don't Make Too Many Changes All at Once

When adopting a new dietary approach like carb cycling, it's essential to make gradual changes. Overhauling your diet overnight can be overwhelming and unsustainable. Here's how to ease into carb cycling for lasting success:

Start Slowly: Begin by incorporating one or two high-carb and low-carb days into your week. A gradual approach allows your body to adjust to the new eating patterns and helps you develop a routine without feeling overwhelmed. As you become more comfortable, you can increase the number of carb-cycling days.

Focus on Small, Achievable Goals: Set small, achievable goals for yourself each week. For example, aim to plan and prepare three healthy meals per week, or try one new recipe each week. These small steps add up over time and help you build sustainable habits.

Monitor and Adjust: Pay attention to how your body responds to carb cycling and make adjustments as needed. If you find certain aspects challenging or notice any adverse effects, tweak your plan to better suit your needs. This could mean adjusting your carb intake, changing your workout routine, or incorporating more flexibility in your meal plans.

Build a Support System

Having a support system can make a significant difference in your carb cycling journey. Surround yourself with people who encourage and support your goals. Here are some ways to build a supportive network:

Share Your Goals: Share your carb cycling goals with friends and family. Explain why you're making these changes and how they can support you. Having people who understand and encourage your efforts can provide motivation and accountability.

Join a Community: Consider joining online communities or local groups focused on health and fitness. These communities can offer valuable advice, support, and motivation. You'll also have the opportunity to share your experiences and learn from others who are on a similar journey.

Work with a Professional: If you're unsure where to start or need personalized guidance, consider working with a nutritionist or dietitian. They can help you create a tailored carb cycling plan that fits your lifestyle and goals, providing expert advice and support along the way.

Adapting Carb Cycling to Life Changes

Life is unpredictable, and your carb cycling plan should be flexible enough to adapt to changes in your circumstances. Here's how to adjust your plan to accommodate life's ups and downs:

Travel: Traveling can disrupt your routine, but with some planning, you can maintain your carb cycling habits on the go. Research restaurants and grocery stores at your destination to find healthy options, pack portable snacks, and stay active while sightseeing, walking, or using hotel gyms.

Busy Schedules: When life gets hectic, it's easy to let your meal planning and workouts slip. Combat this by preparing meals in advance, using time-saving cooking methods like batch cooking and slow cookers, and scheduling your workouts as non-negotiable appointments in your calendar.

Illness or Injury: If you're dealing with an illness or injury, it's essential to listen to your body and prioritize recovery. Adjust your carb cycling plan to accommodate your energy levels and nutritional needs. Focus on gentle, low-impact exercises and nutrient-dense foods that support healing.

Here are additional practical tips to help you make carb cycling a sustainable part of your lifestyle:

• **Keep a Food Diary:** Keeping a food diary can help you stay accountable and track your progress. Record what you eat, how you feel, and any changes you notice in your energy levels, mood, and performance. This can provide valuable insights and help you make informed adjustments to your plan.

• **Stay Hydrated:** Hydration is crucial, especially on low-carb days when you might experience reduced water retention. Drink plenty of water throughout the day to stay hydrated and support your body's functions.

• **Incorporate Mindful Eating:** Practicing mindful eating can enhance your carb cycling experience. Pay attention to your hunger and fullness cues, savor your meals, and avoid distractions while eating. This helps you develop a healthier relationship with food and can prevent overeating.

• **Prepare for Social Situations:** Social situations can sometimes make it challenging to stick to your carb cycling plan. Plan ahead by checking menus in advance, bringing your own healthy options to gatherings, or politely declining foods that don't fit into your plan. Remember, it's okay to enjoy yourself and indulge occasionally, but having a strategy in place can help you stay on track.

Navigating Social Situations

One of the greatest advantages of carb cycling is that you can maintain your social life without sacrificing your dietary goals. Eating out doesn't need to be complicated or stressful if you follow some simple guidelines. Whether you're going to a restaurant, attending a party, or just hanging out with friends, you can stay on track with your nutrition. Let's explore some practical strategies to help you enjoy social occasions while sticking to your carb cycling plan.

Go Out to Eat Like a Pro

Do research beforehand: Preparation is key. Before you head out to a restaurant, take a few minutes to look up their menu online. Almost every restaurant these days has their menu available on their website. Reviewing the menu in advance allows you to game-plan your meal and make informed choices. If you know whether it's a high-carb day, a low-carb day, or a flex day, you can decide which options are best suited for your plan. For instance, if it's a high-carb day, you might look for dishes that include whole grains, legumes, or starchy vegetables. On low-carb days, focus on meals rich in protein and healthy fats, paired with non-starchy vegetables.

Drink water: Staying hydrated is crucial when eating out. Sometimes, what we perceive as hunger is actually thirst. Drinking water before, during, and after your meal helps you avoid mindless snacking and reduces the likelihood of overeating. Water has zero calories, so it's a great way to stay hydrated without adding to your caloric intake. Plus, it aids in digestion and keeps your metabolism functioning efficiently. I always recommend starting your meal with a glass of water and continuing to sip throughout your dining experience.

Sweat it out beforehand: Exercising before you go out to eat can set you up for success. Getting a good workout in, especially a high-intensity interval training (HIIT) session, can boost your metabolism and motivate you to make healthier food choices. When you've worked hard in the gym, you're more likely to want to eat foods that align with your health goals. Exercise also helps manage hunger and cravings, making it easier to stick to your plan when faced with tempting menu options.

Concentrate on real, one-ingredient foods: When choosing meals at a restaurant, try to focus on real, one-ingredient foods. These are foods that haven't been processed or combined with other ingredients, making them healthier options. For example, choose grilled chicken breast, steamed vegetables, or a salad with olive oil and vinegar dressing. Avoid dishes that come with creamy sauces or dressings, as these often contain hidden sugars and unhealthy fats. Don't hesitate to ask how dishes are prepared and request modifications to suit your dietary needs. Most restaurants are happy to accommodate special requests.

Eat slowly: Eating slowly can make a significant difference in how much you eat and how satisfied you feel. When we eat quickly, we often don't give our bodies enough time to register fullness, leading to overeating. Practice mindful eating by taking smaller bites, chewing thoroughly, and savoring each bite. This not only enhances your dining experience but also helps you recognize when you're satisfied, not stuffed. I often remind myself to put my fork down between bites and enjoy the conversation and ambiance.

Additional Tips for Eating Out While Carb Cycling

• **Choose lean proteins:** Opt for lean protein sources like chicken, turkey, fish, or plant-based proteins like tofu and legumes. These options are usually lower in unhealthy fats and can be paired with vegetables for a balanced meal.

• **Load up on vegetables:** Vegetables are your best friend on both high- and low-carb days. They are nutrient-dense, low in calories, and high in fiber, which helps you feel full. Ask for extra veggies on the side instead of starchy sides like fries or rice.

• **Beware of hidden sugars:** Many restaurant dishes, especially sauces and dressings, contain hidden sugars. Opt for vinaigrette dressings or ask for dressings and sauces on the side so you can control the amount you consume.

• **Skip the breadbasket:** The breadbasket is a common pitfall when dining out. It's easy to consume a lot of empty calories before your meal even arrives. Politely decline the breadbasket or ask the server to remove it from the table.

• **Share desserts:** If you're craving something sweet, consider sharing a dessert with a friend. This way, you can enjoy a few bites without consuming too many extra calories. Alternatively, opt for fruit-based desserts, which are generally healthier.

• **Mind your portions:** Restaurant portions can be much larger than what you would typically eat at home. Consider splitting a meal with a dining companion or asking for a to-go box right away and packing up half of your meal to enjoy later.

• **Make smart beverage choices:** Alcohol and sugary drinks can add a lot of calories to your meal. Stick to water, unsweetened tea, or coffee. If you choose to drink alcohol, opt for a glass of wine or a light beer and avoid sugary cocktails.

• **Focus on the social aspect:** Remember that eating out is as much about the social experience as it is about the food. Engage in conversation, enjoy the company, and focus less on the food. This can help you eat more mindfully and enjoy the occasion without overindulging.

Handling Social Gatherings and Events

Social gatherings and events can present unique challenges, but with a little planning, you can handle them successfully:

Offer to bring a dish: If you're attending a potluck or dinner party, offer to bring a dish that fits your carb cycling plan to ensure there will be at least one healthy option available that you can enjoy.

Eat before you go: If you're unsure about the food options available at an event, consider eating a small, healthy meal or snack before you go. This can help curb your hunger and reduce the temptation to indulge in less healthy options.

Scan the buffet: When faced with a buffet, take a walk around and see what's available before filling your plate. This allows you to make informed choices and avoid piling on too much food. Start with vegetables and lean proteins, then add small portions of other items if desired.

Choose your indulgences wisely: If you decide to indulge, choose something that you truly enjoy and savor it. It's better to have a small portion of something you love than to graze on multiple less satisfying options.

Stay hydrated: Just like when dining out, staying hydrated at social events is important. Drink plenty of water to help manage hunger and reduce the likelihood of overeating.

Mind your alcohol intake: Alcohol can lower your inhibitions and lead to overeating. If you choose to drink, do so in moderation and be mindful of the calories in your beverages. Opt for lower-calorie options and alternate with water to stay hydrated.

Remember, it's about balance and making the best choices possible given the circumstances. Stay flexible, be kind to yourself, and enjoy the journey.

Dealing With Hunger and Cravings

Don't let cravings derail your hard work! One of the most challenging aspects of carb cycling—or any dietary change—is managing hunger and cravings. But guess what? There are effective strategies to help you curb those urges and stay on track. Ensuring proper nutrition, managing stress, and getting enough sleep are critical elements for controlling hunger and cravings. Let's dive into some science-based ways to manage your appetite and some healthy alternatives to satisfy common cravings.

Strategies for Managing Hunger

Eat enough protein: Incorporating more protein into your diet can help increase feelings of fullness, reduce hunger hormone levels, and potentially lead to lower calorie intake at subsequent meals. For instance, a study involving 20 overweight or obese adults found that those who had eggs (a high-protein food) for breakfast felt fuller and had lower hunger hormone levels compared to those who ate cereal (a lower-protein food) (Bayham et al., 2014). Another study with 50 overweight adults showed that drinking a high-protein, high-fiber beverage 30 minutes before eating pizza reduced their hunger and the amount of pizza they ate (Sharafi et al., 2018). Protein sources like beans and peas can be just as effective as animal-based proteins in keeping you satisfied. Aim for protein to make up 20–30% of your total calorie intake or consume 0.45–0.55 grams of protein per pound of body weight, although some studies suggest that 0.55–0.73 grams per pound might be more beneficial (Hansen et al., 2021).

Opt for fiber-rich foods: Consuming high-fiber foods helps you feel full by slowing digestion and influencing the release of hormones that increase satiety and regulate appetite. Fiber also helps produce short-chain fatty acids in your gut, which promote fullness. Foods with viscous fibers like pectin, guar gum, and psyllium are particularly filling. A review found that fiber-rich beans, peas, chickpeas, and lentils can increase feelings of fullness by 31% compared to meals without beans. Including fiber-rich whole grains, fruits, vegetables, beans, nuts, and seeds in your diet can promote long-term health and fullness (Li et al., 2014).

Drink plenty of water: Drinking water before meals might suppress hunger and support weight loss. One small study found that people who drank two glasses of water before a meal consumed 22% less food than those who didn't (Corney et al., 2015). Approximately 17 ounces (500 mL) of water may stretch the stomach and send signals of fullness to the brain. Starting your meal with a broth-based soup can have a similar effect, reducing hunger and calorie intake by about 100 calories per meal (Rolls, 2017).

Choose solid foods to tame hunger: Solid foods are more filling than liquids. Solid foods require more chewing, which allows more time for fullness signals to reach the brain and keeps the food in contact with taste buds longer, promoting satiety (Slyper, 2021). Including a variety of textures and flavors in your meals can help you stay satisfied and consume a balanced range of nutrients.

Eat slowly: Eating slowly can help prevent overeating. One study found that people who ate quickly took larger bites and consumed more calories overall, while another study showed that slow eating increased feelings of fullness (McCrickerd & Forde, 2017). Eating slowly allows your body to register satiety signals, helping you feel more satisfied and reduce your overall calorie intake.

Exercise regularly: Regular exercise can help reduce hunger by lowering the activation of brain regions linked to food cravings and increasing feelings of fullness. Both aerobic and resistance exercises are effective, although higher-intensity workouts might have a greater impact on reducing appetite (McNeil et al., 2015). Incorporate physical activities you enjoy into your routine to maximize these benefits.

Get enough sleep: Adequate sleep is essential for managing hunger and preventing weight gain. Studies have shown that a lack of sleep can increase hunger, appetite, and cravings. Sleep deprivation raises levels of ghrelin (a hunger hormone) and lowers levels of leptin (an appetite-regulating hormone) (Yang et al., 2019). Adults generally need 7–9 hours of sleep per night to manage hunger effectively.

Don't deprive yourself: Restricting certain foods can sometimes intensify cravings. Instead, enjoy your favorite foods in moderation. Allowing yourself small portions of foods you crave can be more effective at reducing hunger and cravings than complete deprivation.

Healthy Alternatives for Common Cravings

Craving your favorite comfort foods doesn't have to derail your carb cycling plan. Finding healthy alternatives for the foods you love can help you stay on track without feeling deprived. Here are some practical swaps and tips:

Healthy pizza alternatives: Love pizza? You can still enjoy it by making a few tweaks. Use a whole grain or cauliflower crust instead of traditional dough. Top it with plenty of vegetables, lean proteins, and a moderate amount of cheese. You'll get all the flavors you love without the extra carbs.

Low-carb pasta options: Pasta is another favorite that can be easily adapted. Swap out regular pasta for whole grain, lentil, or chickpea pasta on high-carb days. For low-carb days, try zucchini noodles, spaghetti squash, or shirataki noodles. These alternatives provide similar textures and flavors with fewer carbs. Pro tip: Use a spiralizer for zucchini noodles or roast spaghetti squash and scrape out the strands.

Sweet treats with a twist: If you have a sweet tooth, finding healthier alternatives for desserts can help satisfy your cravings. For high-carb days, enjoy fruits like berries or apples with a dollop of Greek yogurt. On low-carb days, try making desserts with almond flour, coconut flour, or sweeteners like stevia or erythritol.

Black bean for beef burgers: Craving a juicy burger? Try a black bean burger instead. Black beans are high in fiber and protein, promoting gut health while reducing saturated fat intake. Seasoned well, black bean burgers can be just as satisfying as their beef counterparts.

Walnut or cashew cream for heavy cream: For creamy dishes, replace heavy cream with walnut or cashew cream. These alternatives provide unsaturated fats, which help lower bad cholesterol. Blend soaked nuts with water and seasonings for a delicious, creamy substitute.

Cauliflower rice for white rice: Swap nutrient-poor white rice for cauliflower rice. Cauliflower provides a similar texture with added antioxidants and fiber. Pulse cauliflower florets in a food processor and sauté with spices for a nutritious base.

Chia seed jam for jam and jelly: Traditional jams are often loaded with sugar. Make a healthier version by sprinkling chia seeds over warmed berries and letting the mixture thicken. This jam is rich in fiber and omega-3 fatty acids.

Chilled herbal tea for iced sweet tea: Replace sugary iced tea with chilled herbal tea. Hibiscus tea blended with berries offers a naturally sweet, refreshing drink that can help lower blood pressure without the extra calories and sugar.

Coconut aminos for soy sauce: Coconut aminos offer a lower-sodium alternative to soy sauce, providing a similar savory flavor with significantly less salt. Use it to season your dishes for a healthier option.

Crispy chickpeas for croutons: Roasted chickpeas are a crunchy, protein-rich alternative to croutons. They add a satisfying texture to salads while boosting their nutritional value.

Crumbled tofu for ricotta cheese: Tofu can replace ricotta cheese, offering a high-protein, low-fat alternative. Crumble and season tofu to mimic ricotta's texture and flavor in lasagnas, stuffed shells, and other dishes.

"Flax eggs" for eggs: In baking, use "flax eggs" instead of regular eggs. Mix one tablespoon of ground flaxseeds with three tablespoons of water and let it rest until it thickens. This mixture binds ingredients without the cholesterol of eggs.

Jicama wraps for corn tortillas: Jicama wraps are a crunchy, low-carb alternative to corn tortillas. High in fiber and antioxidants, jicama wraps can be used for tacos and wraps. Slice jicama thinly for a fresh, crisp shell.

Nutritional yeast for parmesan cheese: Nutritional yeast is a vegan alternative to Parmesan cheese. It's rich in protein and contains all nine essential amino acids. Sprinkle it over pasta, salads, and roasted vegetables for a cheesy flavor without the added fats.

Seasoned shredded jackfruit for shredded meats: Jackfruit is a versatile fruit that can mimic the texture of shredded meats. When well-seasoned, it works well as a substitute for pulled pork or chicken, offering a nutritious option with vitamin A and other nutrients.

Wheat bread for white bread: Switch from white bread to whole wheat bread to increase your fiber intake and get more nutrients. Whole-wheat bread contains more vitamins and minerals than refined white bread, supporting overall health.

Staying Motivated and Consistent

Maintaining motivation and consistency is one of the most significant hurdles in any carb cycling journey. To reach your weight loss goals, it's essential to stay committed and not take shortcuts. Remember, you're in control, and with the right strategies, you can stay on track. Let's explore some effective ways to keep yourself accountable and motivated.

Set achievable goals: Setting realistic and attainable goals is crucial. Aim to lose around 10 percent of your weight within six months and focus on maintaining that loss for over a year. Instead of obsessing over the number on the scale, concentrate on behavior changes such as reducing your daily fat intake or cutting out sugary snacks. Setting non-weight-related goals, like training for a 5K, can also be beneficial. The weight loss that comes as a result will feel like a bonus and provide additional motivation.

Create a plan that fits your lifestyle: Develop a weight-loss plan that seamlessly integrates into your daily life. Small changes, like cutting 150 calories a day, can result in significant long-term weight loss. Modify your current eating habits by downsizing portions or preparing foods differently. Tailor your plan to include foods you enjoy and can't live without, ensuring you don't feel deprived. If you enjoy snacking, consider having several mini meals throughout the day.

Document your plan: Writing down your weight loss plan is vital for success. List all the reasons for losing weight and define your motivation. Once you have a clear goal, create a detailed monthly action plan with specific and realistic targets. This approach will help you stay focused and track your progress.

Honor your commitments: Struggling to maintain motivation? Practice integrity in other areas of your life to build confidence in your ability to achieve your weight-loss goals. Pay off debts, fulfill promises to friends and family, and organize your environment. By keeping commitments in various aspects of life, you strengthen your belief in your ability to stick to your weight loss plan.

Avoid comparisons: Comparing yourself to unrealistic standards can hinder your progress. Instead of looking at images of supermodels, find inspiration in your own healthy moments. Displaying pictures of yourself at your best can provide a positive and realistic source of motivation.

Focus on how you feel: Shift your focus from numbers on the scale to how you feel after healthy meals or workouts. Concentrating on the positive emotions associated with these activities can enhance your motivation to continue.

Celebrate small wins: Don't wait until you reach your final goal to reward yourself. Celebrate small milestones along the way with meaningful rewards. This could be anything from a pedicure after hitting a minor target to a day at the spa when you reach a significant milestone. Rewards reinforce positive behavior and keep you motivated.

Visualize your success: Hang a piece of clothing you aspire to wear by your mirror as a daily reminder of your goals. Visualizing yourself in that outfit can provide a daily dose of motivation to stay on track.

Team up for support: Joining forces with a friend or a group can significantly boost your motivation. Studies have shown that social influence in team-based weight-loss competitions can lead to more substantial results than going solo. Having a workout buddy or a support group makes the journey more enjoyable and keeps you accountable.

Clarify your motivations: Understanding your core motivations is essential for staying driven. Identify what inspires you and focus on those aspects. For example, if staying active in your children's lives is a priority, remind yourself how exercise and healthy eating contribute to that goal.

Seek professional guidance: Finding the right balance of healthy foods that keep you satisfied can be challenging. Consider consulting a dietitian or nutritionist for personalized advice. If motivation issues are linked to feelings of depression or anxiety, speaking with a therapist can be beneficial.

Limit weigh-ins: While the scale can be a helpful tool, weighing yourself too frequently can be counterproductive. Instead, weigh yourself once a week or every two weeks to monitor progress. Focus on non-scale victories to maintain motivation and track your success.

Keep a photo journal: Documenting your journey through photos can provide visual evidence of your progress. Take pictures after workouts or healthy meals to capture changes in your lifestyle and body. Reviewing these photos can offer a motivational boost.

Silence negative self-talk: Self-criticism can sabotage your efforts. When you catch yourself being overly critical, take a moment to pause and refocus. Practice self-compassion and recognize your achievements, no matter how small.

Practice positive self-talk: Shift your focus from self-criticism to self-appreciation. Recognize and be grateful for what your body can do. Focus on functionality rather than appearance to cultivate a positive mindset.

Surround yourself with positivity: Create an environment that reflects your healthy lifestyle goals. Stock your fridge with healthy foods, display fruits on the counter, and keep your exercise equipment accessible. Adjusting your surroundings can make it easier to stay on track.

Utilize technology: Take advantage of weight-loss apps and other technological tools to stay motivated. These apps can help you find recipes, track progress, and connect with support communities. Keeping your motivation mobile can make it easier to stick to your plan.

Get friends involved: Rewarding yourself can be more fun with friends. Ask friends to buy and wrap small gifts for you to open when you reach specific milestones. This adds an element of surprise and joy to your journey.

Set non-scale goals: Sometimes the scale doesn't reflect your efforts, but that doesn't mean you're not making progress. Set goals related to fitness or healthy eating, and celebrate these achievements. Focusing on non-scale victories can keep you motivated when the numbers aren't moving.

You need to keep in mind that motivation naturally fluctuates, and it's okay to have off days. The key is to keep going and use these strategies to stay on track.

We've all faced those moments of doubt and temptation where giving up seems like the easier option. But every step you take, no matter how small, brings you closer to your goals. Staying motivated isn't about always feeling inspired; it's about pushing through even when you don't feel like it.

The strategies we've discussed—setting achievable goals, creating a personalized plan, documenting your journey, celebrating small victories, and surrounding yourself with a supportive environment—are all designed to keep you moving forward. There will be days when you're full of energy and enthusiasm, and other days when you feel like you're dragging yourself along. Accept these natural rhythms and use them to your advantage. Remember, you don't need your motivation tank to be full to make progress; you just need to keep it from running empty.

When you hit a rough patch, take a break, refocus, and remind yourself why you started this journey in the first place. Celebrate every small win, be it a healthier food choice, a completed workout, or even resisting a craving. These moments add up and reinforce your commitment. And don't forget the power of support—whether it's a friend, a family member, or a group of like-minded individuals, having someone to share your journey with can make all the difference.

As we transition to the next chapter, we'll dive deeper into expert tactics for optimal results. Here, you'll learn advanced strategies to fine-tune your carb cycling plan, ensuring you achieve the best possible outcomes. These expert tips will help you overcome plateaus, maximize your efforts, and maintain your progress for the long haul. Stay with me, and let's continue this journey together, building on your successes and pushing toward your ultimate goals.

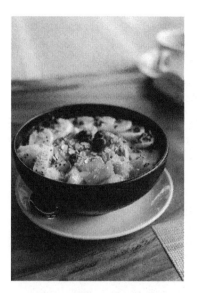

Chapter Seven

Expert Tactics for Optimal Results

You've already laid a solid foundation by understanding the basics of carb cycling and overcoming initial hurdles, now, it's time to refine your approach and maximize your results. Trust me, the effort you put in here will pay off significantly!

One of the most common challenges people face is hitting a fat loss plateau. It's frustrating when you've been working hard, and the progress seems to stall. Don't worry; we'll arm you with the tactics you need to break through those barriers. You can reignite your fat-burning engine by tweaking your carb cycling routine and making small adjustments. We'll explore the science behind plateaus and provide actionable steps to overcome them.

We're also going to discuss how to combine intermittent fasting with carb cycling. This powerful duo can enhance your results by optimizing your metabolism and improving your body's efficiency when using energy.

I'll guide you through the process, ensuring you understand how to implement this strategy safely and effectively. You'll learn about different fasting windows and how to align them with your carb cycling days for maximum impact.

Another critical aspect we'll cover is the effective use of supplementation. While whole foods should always be your primary source of nutrients, supplements can play a supportive role in filling any nutritional gaps. We'll look at which supplements can enhance your carb cycling efforts, from protein powders to vitamins and minerals. I'll help you make sense of the overwhelming world of supplements so you can make informed choices that align with your goals.

To make all of this practical, we'll set the stage for a 7-day diet and exercise plan. This plan is designed to kickstart your journey, offering a structured approach to applying the advanced strategies you'll learn. Aiming to break a plateau, boost your performance, or accelerate fat loss? This plan will provide a clear path forward.

Get ready to elevate your carb cycling game! These expert tactics are here to help you achieve optimal results and sustain your progress.

Carb Cycling for Fat Loss Plateaus

Hitting a plateau in your fat-loss journey can be incredibly frustrating. You've been diligent with your carb cycling, following your plan to the letter, and yet the scale refuses to budge. This stagnant phase can be discouraging, but understanding what a plateau is and how to identify it is the first step toward overcoming it. Let's discuss what plateaus are and how you can recognize them.

What Is a Plateau?

A plateau occurs when your body adapts to your current diet and exercise regimen, causing your weight loss to stall. It's a period where, despite continuing your efforts, you no longer see progress on the scale or in your body measurements. Plateaus are a natural part of the weight-loss process and can happen to anyone (Cronkleton, 2022). They occur because our bodies are incredibly efficient at adapting to changes in diet and exercise. When you first start carb cycling, your body responds well to the new approach, and you likely see significant progress. However, over time, your body adjusts to this new normal, and the initial calorie deficit or metabolic boost you experienced starts to diminish.

The science behind plateaus involves a combination of metabolic adaptation, hormonal changes, and energy balance. Metabolic adaptation, also known as adaptive thermogenesis, refers to the process by which your body becomes more efficient at using energy. Essentially, your metabolism slows down to conserve energy, making it harder to continue losing weight. This is a survival mechanism that helped our ancestors survive during times of food scarcity (Cronkleton, 2022).

Hormonal changes also play a significant role in plateaus. When you're in a calorie deficit, levels of leptin, a hormone that regulates hunger and metabolism, decrease. Lower leptin levels signal your brain to conserve energy and increase hunger, making it more challenging to stick to your diet. Additionally, other hormones like thyroid hormones, which regulate metabolism, can also decrease during prolonged dieting, further slowing your metabolic rate.

How to Identify a Plateau

Recognizing a plateau requires paying close attention to various indicators of progress. Here are some common signs that you might be experiencing a plateau:

Stable weight: One of the most obvious signs of a plateau is when your weight remains the same for an extended period of time, typically several weeks. If you're consistently sticking to your carb cycling plan and exercise routine but not seeing any changes on the scale, you might be on a plateau.

Consistent measurements: In addition to weight, taking regular body measurements can provide insight into your progress. If your measurements (waist, hips, thighs, etc.) have stalled alongside your weight, it's another indicator that you might be on a plateau.

Clothing fit: Sometimes, the scale might not move, but your clothes might fit differently. However, if you notice that your clothes are fitting the same way they have for weeks, it's a sign that you might be on a plateau.

Body fat percentage: Tracking your body fat percentage can be more telling than weight alone. If your body fat percentage remains unchanged despite your efforts, it's likely that you've hit a plateau.

Performance metrics: Pay attention to your performance in the gym or during your workouts. If you're not seeing improvements in strength, endurance, or other fitness metrics, it could indicate a plateau.

Mental and physical fatigue: Experiencing increased fatigue, both mentally and physically, can be a sign of a plateau. This fatigue can result from your body adapting to your current regimen, signaling that it's time for a change.

Tools to Identify a Plateau

Using various tools can help you identify whether you're on a plateau. Here are some methods to consider:

• **Scale:** Regularly weighing yourself can help track your progress over time. However, it's essential to remember that weight can fluctuate daily due to various factors like water retention, muscle gain, and food intake. Look for trends over several weeks rather than focusing on daily changes.

• **Measurements:** Use a tape measure to track the circumference of different body parts, such as your waist, hips, and thighs. Taking measurements every two weeks can provide a clearer picture of your progress.

• **Body fat analysis:** Tools like calipers, bioelectrical impedance scales, or DEXA scans can help track changes in body fat percentage. While some methods are more accurate than others, consistently using the same method can help you monitor trends.

• **Progress photos:** Taking regular progress photos can provide a visual record of your changes. Sometimes, visual changes might not be apparent on the scale or in measurements but can be seen in photos.

• **Fitness tracking:** Monitoring your workout performance, such as the weight you lift, the distance you run, or your overall endurance, can help identify plateaus. If you're not seeing improvements or if your performance has stalled, it could be a sign that you've hit a plateau.

Psychological Aspects of Plateaus

Understanding the psychological aspects of plateaus is also crucial. It's easy to become discouraged when progress stalls, but maintaining a positive mindset is vital. Here are some tips to help you stay motivated:

Patience: Remember that plateaus are a normal part of the weight-loss journey. Stay patient and understand that your body needs time to adjust.

Focus on non-scale victories: Celebrate achievements that aren't related to the scale, such as improved fitness levels, better mood, increased energy, and healthier eating habits.

Reflect on your journey: Take time to reflect on how far you've come. Remind yourself of the progress you've made and the positive changes in your lifestyle.

Seek support: Sharing your experiences with a support group or a friend can provide encouragement and motivation. Talking about your frustrations may help you gain perspective and renew your commitment.

Adjust your goals: Reassess and adjust your goals if necessary. Sometimes, shifting your focus to new objectives can reignite your motivation and help you overcome the plateau.

Common Misconceptions About Plateaus

There are several misconceptions about plateaus that can lead to unnecessary frustration:

• **Plateaus mean failure:** A common misconception is that hitting a plateau means you're failing. In reality, plateaus are a natural part of the process and indicate that your body is adapting.

• **Weight loss should be linear:** Many people expect weight loss to be a continuous downward trend. However, weight loss often involves fluctuations, and plateaus are a normal part of this journey.

• **More exercise equals faster progress:** While exercise is essential, more isn't always better. Overtraining can lead to burnout and slow progress. It's important to find a balance that works for your body.

• **Cutting more calories is the solution:** Drastically cutting calories can be counterproductive and lead to further metabolic slowdown. It's essential to fuel your body adequately and make gradual adjustments.

Identifying a plateau is the first step in overcoming it. Understanding what a plateau is and recognizing the signs can help you take proactive steps to get back on track. Now, let's discuss effective strategies to break through plateaus, ensuring you have the tools and knowledge to overcome these challenges and continue your journey to optimal health.

How to Overcome Plateaus

So, before you throw in the towel, let's explore how you can overcome these plateaus and get back on track.

Dial down your workouts: It might sound counterintuitive, but sometimes less is more. Overly intense workouts can lead to exhaustion and stress, which can hinder weight loss. Aim for moderate-intensity aerobic activities like brisk walking, light biking, swimming, or controlled strength training. The Department of Health and Human Services recommends at least 150 minutes of moderate-intensity aerobic activity per week, along with strength training twice a week (Physical Activity Guidelines for Americans, 2018). Taking this balanced approach can prevent burnout and promote sustainable weight loss.

Increase protein intake: Adding more protein to your diet can help overcome hunger and keep you feeling full longer. Protein has a higher thermic effect than fats and carbohydrates, meaning your body burns more calories by digesting it. Aim to include protein-rich foods like beans, lean meats, fish, eggs, and dairy in your meals. This can help you maintain muscle mass while losing fat, boosting your metabolic rate.

Manage stress: Chronic stress can elevate cortisol levels, leading to weight gain or stalled weight loss. Incorporate stress-reducing activities like yoga, meditation, or even a relaxing bath into your routine. Being aware of weight-loss plateaus and cutting yourself some slack can also help reduce stress.

Keep a food journal: Tracking what you eat can help you stay accountable and identify areas where you might be slipping. A food journal allows you to see your eating patterns and make necessary adjustments. Research shows that people who keep food diaries tend to lose more weight than those who don't (Hollis et al., 2008).

Prioritize strength training: While cardio is great for burning calories, strength training is crucial for maintaining and building muscle mass. Muscle tissue burns more calories at rest than fat tissue, so increasing your muscle mass can boost your metabolic rate. Aim for at least two strength training sessions per week to keep your metabolism active.

Increase daily activity: Beyond structured workouts, increasing your daily activity can help overcome a plateau. Simple changes like taking the stairs, walking during breaks, or doing household chores can increase your overall calorie burn. Remember, every little bit helps.

Limit alcohol consumption: Alcohol can contribute to weight gain and plateaus by lowering your blood sugar and inhibiting fat burning. Try to limit your alcohol intake to two or three drinks per week and opt for drinking with meals to stabilize your blood sugar.

Be mindful of "healthy" foods: Certain foods with a health halo, like nuts, granola, and full-fat dairy, can be high in calories. While they are nutritious, consuming them in large quantities can stall your weight loss. Practice portion control and enjoy these foods in moderation.

Increase fiber intake: Fiber helps you feel full longer and supports healthy digestion. Incorporate high-fiber foods like lentils, black beans, avocados, and whole grains into your diet. These foods can help manage hunger and support weight loss.

Incorporate HIIT workouts: High-Intensity Interval Training (HIIT) involves short bursts of intense activity followed by rest periods. HIIT can help break through plateaus by shocking your body and increasing calorie burn. Adding sprints or jumping jacks to your routine can make your workouts more effective.

Stay hydrated: Drinking enough water is crucial for weight loss. Sometimes, thirst can be mistaken for hunger, leading to unnecessary snacking. Keep a water bottle with you throughout the day and aim to drink at least eight glasses of water daily.

Add more vegetables to your meals: Vegetables are low in calories and high in fiber, making them perfect for weight loss. Aim to include vegetables at every meal to increase your fiber intake and help you feel full. This can also ensure you get a variety of nutrients to support your overall health.

Incorporate probiotics: A healthy gut can aid in weight loss. Probiotics found in fermented foods like kimchi, sauerkraut, and yogurt can support a healthy gut microbiome. If fermented foods aren't your thing, consider taking a probiotic supplement.

Ensure adequate sleep: Sleep is essential for overall health and weight loss. Studies show that a lack of sleep can lead to weight gain and make it harder to lose weight. Aim for 7-9 hours of sleep per night and establish a consistent sleep routine. Creating a bedtime ritual, such as turning off screens and keeping your room cool, can improve your sleep quality.

Breaking Plateaus with Carb Cycling

Carb cycling itself can be an effective tool to overcome weight loss plateaus. By alternating between high-carb and low-carb days, you can prevent your body from adapting to a single routine. Here are some tips on how to use carb cycling to break through plateaus:

• **Adjust carb ratios:** If you've been following a specific carb ratio, try tweaking it slightly. Increase your carb intake on high-carb days or decrease it on low-carb days to keep your body guessing.

• **Incorporate re-feed days:** Re-feed days, where you temporarily increase your carb intake, can boost leptin levels and reset your metabolism. Plan a re-feed day once a week to jumpstart your weight loss.

• **Vary your carb sources:** Mix up your carb sources to include a variety of whole grains, fruits, and vegetables. This can prevent monotony and ensure you get a range of nutrients.

• **Combine with intermittent fasting:** Pairing carb cycling with intermittent fasting can enhance fat loss. Try incorporating a fasting window, such as 16/8, where you fast for 16 hours and eat during an 8-hour window. Align your high-carb days with your most active days for optimal results.

• **Track your progress:** Keep a detailed log of your carb cycling routine, including what you eat and how you feel. This can help you identify patterns and make the necessary adjustments.

• **Stay flexible:** Listen to your body and be willing to adapt your carb cycling plan as needed. What works for one person might not work for another, so find what suits you best.

Intermittent Fasting and Carb Cycling

Let's cut straight to the chase: intermittent fasting is a game-changer. If you've been on the fence about trying it, or if you're curious about how it works, this is the place to start. Intermittent fasting (IF) isn't just another diet fad; it's a powerful tool that can complement your carb cycling journey and supercharge your weight loss efforts. So, let's dive into what intermittent fasting is, how it works, and why it might be the missing piece in your fitness puzzle.

What Is Intermittent Fasting?

Intermittent fasting is an eating pattern that alternates between periods of eating and fasting. Unlike traditional diets that focus on what you eat, IF focuses on when you eat. The idea is simple: by restricting your eating window, you give your body more time to burn fat and repair itself (Gunnars, 2024). There are several different approaches to intermittent fasting, but they all revolve around this fundamental principle of cycling between periods of eating and fasting.

Different Methods of Intermittent Fasting

There are various ways to implement intermittent fasting, and the best method for you will depend on your lifestyle, preferences, and goals. Here are some of the most popular approaches (Snyder & Gunnars, 2023):

• **16/8 method:** This is one of the most common and straightforward methods. You fast for 16 hours each day and eat all your meals within an 8-hour window. For example, you might eat between noon and 8 p.m. and fast from 8 p.m. to noon the next day. This method is popular because it's relatively easy to stick to and can be adjusted to fit most schedules.

• **5:2 diet:** With this approach, you eat normally for five days of the week and significantly reduce your calorie intake (about 500–600 calories) on the other two days. These two fasting days can be non-consecutive, such as Monday and Thursday, allowing you to maintain a more regular eating pattern on the other days.

• **Eat-stop-eat:** This method involves fasting for a full 24 hours once or twice a week. For example, you might stop eating after dinner at 7 p.m. and not eat again until 7 p.m. the next day. This can be more challenging than the 16/8 method, but it can also provide significant benefits.

• **Alternate day fasting:** As the name suggests, you alternate between days of normal eating and days of fasting. On fasting days, you may consume very few calories or none at all. This method can be quite effective, but it is also more rigorous.

• **Warrior diet:** This involves eating small amounts of raw fruits and vegetables during the day and having one large meal at night. Typically, this eating window is around 4 hours, with a 20-hour fasting period.

How Intermittent Fasting Works

The science behind intermittent fasting is truly fascinating. When you eat, your body spends several hours processing and absorbing food, using it for immediate energy, and storing the rest as fat. During a fast, your insulin levels drop, signaling your body to start burning stored fat for energy. Let's take a closer look at the key biological processes at play during intermittent fasting.

Insulin Sensitivity

Insulin is a hormone produced by the pancreas that allows your body to use or store glucose (sugar) from carbohydrates in the food you eat. When you consume food, your blood sugar levels rise, prompting your pancreas to release insulin. This insulin helps cells absorb glucose to be used for energy or stored as fat for later use.

During periods of fasting, insulin levels drop significantly because there is no incoming food to process. Lower insulin levels are crucial for fat burning because they make stored body fat more accessible as an energy source. Without the constant presence of insulin, your body can tap into its fat reserves, converting stored fat into energy, which is essential for weight loss (Yuan et al., 2022).

Increased insulin sensitivity means your body requires less insulin to process glucose, which is beneficial for your overall metabolic health. High insulin sensitivity can prevent conditions like insulin resistance, which is a precursor to type 2 diabetes.

Human Growth Hormone (HGH)

Human Growth Hormone (HGH) plays a vital role in growth, metabolism, and muscle repair. During fasting, the secretion of HGH can increase dramatically—sometimes by as much as fivefold. This spike in HGH levels is beneficial for several reasons (Mawer, 2023):

• **Fat loss:** HGH helps in the breakdown of fat and its conversion into energy, making it easier for the body to burn fat during fasting periods.

• **Muscle gain:** Higher levels of HGH support the maintenance and growth of lean muscle mass, which is crucial for a healthy metabolism. Muscle tissue burns more calories than fat tissue, even at rest, contributing to a higher metabolic rate.

• **Metabolism boost:** By promoting muscle growth and fat loss, HGH helps boost your overall metabolism, making it easier to achieve and maintain a healthy weight.

Cellular Repair

One of the most remarkable benefits of intermittent fasting is its impact on cellular repair processes, particularly autophagy. Autophagy is the body's way of cleaning out damaged cells to regenerate newer, healthier cells. During fasting, the body initiates autophagy, which involves breaking down and recycling old, dysfunctional cellular components.

This cellular "clean-up" process has several significant benefits (Gunnars, 2023):

• **Improved health:** By removing damaged cells, autophagy can reduce the risk of developing various diseases, including cancer, Alzheimer's disease, and other age-related conditions.

• **Reduced inflammation:** Autophagy helps to clear out cellular debris and reduce inflammation, which is linked to many chronic diseases.

• **Longevity:** Enhanced cellular repair and reduced inflammation contribute to overall health and longevity, potentially extending lifespan.

Gene Expression

Fasting influences the expression of several genes and molecules involved in longevity and disease protection. These changes can enhance the body's ability to handle stress and improve overall health. Some of the key changes in gene expression include (Deota et al., 2023):

• **Stress resistance:** Fasting increases the production of proteins that enhance the body's ability to cope with stress. These proteins help repair DNA, support immune function, and protect cells from damage.

• **Anti-aging:** Intermittent fasting activates certain pathways that promote longevity. For example, it can increase the expression of sirtuins (SIRTs), a group of proteins that regulate cellular health and are associated with lifespan extension.

• **Metabolic health:** Fasting improves the expression of genes involved in metabolism, enhancing the body's ability to regulate blood sugar levels and process fats.

When you combine these biological processes, it becomes clear why intermittent fasting is such a powerful tool for weight loss and overall health. By allowing your body to lower insulin levels, increase HGH production, enhance cellular repair, and improve gene expression, you create an optimal environment for fat burning and metabolic health.

Benefits of Intermittent Fasting

Intermittent fasting offers a host of benefits beyond weight loss. Here are some of the key advantages (Kandola & French, 2023):

Weight loss and fat loss: By reducing your eating window, you naturally consume fewer calories. Coupled with increased fat burning, this can lead to significant weight loss. Studies have shown that intermittent fasting can be as effective, if not more so, than traditional calorie-restricted diets.

Improved metabolic health: Intermittent fasting can improve various metabolic markers, including blood sugar levels, insulin sensitivity, and lipid profiles. This can lower your risk of type 2 diabetes and heart disease.

Enhanced brain function: Fasting has been shown to improve brain health by reducing oxidative stress and inflammation and promoting the growth of new neurons. It may also lower the risk of neurodegenerative diseases like Alzheimer's.

Simplicity and flexibility: One of the greatest benefits of intermittent fasting is its simplicity. There are no complicated meal plans or special foods required. You simply eat within your designated window and fast the rest of the time.

Potential longevity: Intermittent fasting can extend lifespans (Haseltine, 2023). While more research is needed on humans, improvements in metabolic health and reduced risk of chronic diseases are promising indicators.

If you're new to intermittent fasting, here are some tips to help you get started:

• **Start gradually:** Begin with a shorter fasting window, like 12 hours, and gradually increase it as you become more comfortable. This can make the transition easier and more sustainable.

• **Stay hydrated:** Drink plenty of water during your fasting period to stay hydrated and help manage hunger.

• **Eat nutrient-dense foods:** Focus on whole, nutrient-dense foods during your eating window to ensure you're getting the vitamins and minerals your body needs.

• **Plan your meals:** Having a plan can make intermittent fasting easier. Know what you'll eat when your fasting period ends to avoid impulsive, unhealthy choices.

• **Pay attention to your body:** Pay attention to how your body responds to fasting. If you feel dizzy, excessively fatigued, or unwell, it might be a sign that you need to adjust your approach.

• **Be patient:** It might take some time for your body to adapt to intermittent fasting. Give yourself a few weeks to adjust before evaluating its effectiveness.

Potential Challenges and How to Overcome Them

While intermittent fasting offers many benefits, it's not without its challenges. Here are some common hurdles and how to overcome them:

Hunger: It's normal to feel hungry when you first start fasting. Drinking water, tea, or black coffee can help manage hunger. Over time, your body will adjust, and hunger pangs will decrease.

Social situations: Fasting can be tricky in social settings. Try to plan your fasting schedule around social events or communicate your goals with friends and family so they can support you.

Energy levels: Some people might experience low energy levels initially. Ensure you're eating balanced, nutrient-dense meals during your eating window to keep your energy up.

Overeating: It's easy to overeat during your eating window if you're overly hungry. Stick to a meal plan and focus on portion control to avoid this pitfall.

Mindset: Fasting requires a mental shift. Viewing it as a positive lifestyle choice rather than a restrictive diet can help maintain a healthy relationship with food.

Intermittent fasting is a powerful tool that, when combined with carb cycling, can significantly enhance your weight loss and overall health.

Combining Intermittent Fasting with Carb Cycling

Now, let's talk about combining intermittent fasting with carb cycling. Each of these strategies is powerful on its own, but when you combine them, you create a synergy that can supercharge your weight loss and overall health. Trust me, this combo can be a game-changer.

Why Combine Intermittent Fasting with Carb Cycling?

The primary reason to combine intermittent fasting (IF) with carb cycling is to maximize fat burning while maintaining muscle mass and boosting overall metabolic health. Both IF and carb cycling target insulin sensitivity, fat utilization, and metabolic efficiency, but they do so in complementary ways. Here's a closer look at the benefits:

Enhanced fat burning: Intermittent fasting helps lower insulin levels and increases human growth hormone, making it easier for your body to access and burn stored fat. Carb cycling, with its alternating high and low carb days, prevents your metabolism from becoming too efficient at storing fat, keeping your body in a fat-burning mode.

Muscle preservation: While fasting periods and low-carb days promote fat burning, high-carb days in carb cycling help replenish glycogen stores and provide the necessary fuel for muscle growth and recovery. This balance ensures you're not sacrificing muscle mass while losing weight.

Improved insulin sensitivity: Both strategies improve insulin sensitivity, reducing the risk of insulin resistance and type 2 diabetes. By keeping insulin levels low during fasting and alternating carb intake, you optimize your body's ability to process and use carbohydrates effectively.

Increased flexibility and adherence: Combining these two methods allows for greater dietary flexibility. You're not stuck in a rigid eating plan, making it easier to stick with your regimen long-term. This flexibility can enhance adherence, a crucial factor for sustained success.

How to Combine Intermittent Fasting with Carb Cycling

Combining intermittent fasting with carb cycling might seem complex at first, but it's all about planning and finding a routine that fits your lifestyle. Here's a step-by-step guide to help you get started:

Step 1: Choose your intermittent fasting method

First, decide which intermittent fasting method works best for you. The 16/8 method is a great starting point for most people, as it's relatively easy to maintain and fits well with a typical daily schedule. Here's a quick refresher on the popular IF methods:

• *16/8 method:* Fast for 16 hours and eat within an 8-hour window. For example, you might eat between noon and 8 p.m. and fast from 8 p.m. to noon the next day.

• *5:2 diet:* Eat normally for five days and reduce calorie intake to 500–600 calories on two non-consecutive days.

• *Eat-stop-eat:* Fast for a full 24 hours once or twice a week.

• *Alternate-day fasting:* Alternate between days of regular eating and fasting or very low-calorie intake.

• *Warrior diet:* Eat small amounts of raw fruits and vegetables during the day and have one large meal at night.

Choose the method that aligns best with your daily routine and preferences.

Step 2: Plan your carb cycling schedule

Next, outline your carb cycling plan. Determine your high-carb and low-carb days based on your activity levels and goals. Here's a basic framework:

> **High-carb days:** Typically scheduled on days with intense workouts or higher activity levels. These days replenish glycogen stores, support muscle recovery, and provide energy for performance. Aim for 50–60% of your daily calories from carbohydrates.

Low-carb days: Scheduled on rest days or days with light activity. These days, they encourage fat burning by keeping insulin levels low. Aim for 10–20% of your daily calories from carbohydrates.

Moderate-carb days (optional): These can be included to provide a balanced approach on days with moderate activity. Aim for 30–40% of your daily calories from carbohydrates.

Step 3: Align fasting windows with carb days

Now, align your fasting windows with your carb cycling schedule for maximum effectiveness. Here's how:

High-carb days: Plan your eating window around your most active times. For example, if you workout in the evening, start your eating window a few hours before your workout to fuel your performance and recovery. A typical schedule might look like this:
• Fast from 8 p.m. to noon the next day.
• Eating window from noon to 8 p.m., with a focus on high-carb meals.

Low-carb days: Extend your fasting window to maximize fat burning. Since low-carb days are typically on rest days or light activity days, you can afford to fast a bit longer. A typical schedule might look like this:
• Fast from 8 p.m. to 2 p.m. the next day.
• Eating window from 2 p.m. to 8 p.m., with a focus on low-carb, high-protein meals.

Step 4: Optimize meal timing and composition

Meal timing and composition are crucial for optimizing the benefits of both intermittent fasting and carb cycling. Here's a breakdown of what to eat and when:

• *Pre-workout nutrition (high-carb days):* Have a balanced meal 2–3 hours before your workout, including a good mix of complex carbohydrates, lean protein, and healthy fats. This fuels your workout and ensures you have enough energy to perform at your best. For example: Grilled chicken with quinoa and steamed vegetables.

• *Post-workout nutrition (high-carb days):* Eat a high-carb, high-protein meal within 2 hours post-workout to replenish glycogen stores and kick-start muscle recovery. For example: A smoothie with protein powder, banana, spinach, and almond milk.

• *Meals on low-carb days:* Focus on high-protein, moderate-fat meals with plenty of non-starchy vegetables. This helps keep insulin levels low and promotes fat burning. For example: Baked salmon with avocado and a side of mixed greens.

• *Hydration:* Stay hydrated throughout your fasting period and eating window. Drink plenty of water, herbal teas, and black coffee (if you enjoy it) to keep hunger at bay and support overall health.

Step 5: Adjust based on feedback

Your body will provide feedback on how it's responding to this combined approach. Pay attention to how you feel, your energy levels, and your progress. Here are some tips for making adjustments:

• *Track your progress:* Keep a journal to log your meals, workouts, and how you feel each day. Note any changes in weight, measurements, or performance.

• *Find your balance:* If you feel excessively fatigued or hungry, consider adjusting your fasting window or carb intake. The goal is to find a balance that works for you.

• *Stay flexible:* Don't be afraid to tweak your plan. If a certain fasting window or carb cycling pattern isn't working, try a different approach. Flexibility is key to long-term success.

Step 6: Overcome common challenges

Combining intermittent fasting with carb cycling can present some challenges, but with the right strategies, you can overcome them. Here are some common issues and solutions:

• *Hunger during fasting:* Hunger is natural, especially when you first start fasting. Stay hydrated and consume fiber-rich, nutrient-dense foods during your eating window to help manage hunger.

• *Social situations:* Social events can be tricky. Plan ahead by checking the menu if you're eating out and adjust your fasting and carb cycling schedule to accommodate these events. Communicate your goals with friends and family for support.

• *Energy levels:* If you experience low energy, ensure you're eating balanced meals with adequate protein, healthy fats, and carbs during your eating window. Adjust your fasting window if necessary.

• *Plateaus:* If you hit a plateau, revisit your plan, and make adjustments. Sometimes small tweaks, like changing your carb intake or modifying your fasting schedule, can make a big difference.

A Week with Intermittent Fasting and Carb Cycling

To give you a concrete idea, here's an example of how you might structure a week by combining intermittent fasting with carb cycling:

Day	Carb Level & Fasting Windows	Lunch	Snack	Dinner
Monday	High-Carb Fasting window: 8:00 p.m. (Sunday) to noon Eating window: Noon to 8:00 p.m.	• Grilled chicken • Quinoa • Sweet potatoes • Mixed greens	• Greek yogurt • Berries	• Whole grain pasta • Marinara sauce • Lean ground turkey • Side salad
Tuesday	Low-Carb Fasting window: 8:00 p.m. (Monday) to 2:00 p.m. Eating window: 2:00 p.m. to 8:00 p.m.	• Baked salmon • Avocado • Mixed greens	• Handful of nuts	• Chicken stir-fry • Broccoli • Bell peppers • Side of cauliflower rice
Wednesday	Moderate-Carb Fasting window: 8:00 p.m. (Tuesday) to noon Eating window: Noon to 8:00 p.m.	• Turkey and vegetable wrap • Whole grain tortilla	• Apple • Almond butter	• Grilled shrimp • Brown rice • Steamed vegetables
Thursday	High-Carb Fasting window: 8:00 p.m. (Wednesday) to noon Eating window: Noon to 8:00 p.m.	• Quinoa salad • Chickpeas • Cucumbers • Tomatoes • Feta	• Protein smoothie • Banana • Spinach • Almond milk	• Beef stir-fry • Mixed vegetables • Jasmine rice

Day	Carb Level & Fasting Windows	Lunch	Snack	Dinner
Friday	Low-Carb Fasting window: 8:00 p.m. (Thursday) to 2:00 p.m. Eating window: 2:00 p.m. to 8:00 p.m.	• Tuna salad • Mixed greens • Olives • Olive oil dressing	• Celery sticks • Hummus	• Grilled chicken • Zucchini noodles • Pesto
Saturday	Moderate-Carb Fasting window: 8:00 p.m. (Friday) to 2:00 p.m. Eating window: 2:00 p.m. to 8:00 p.m.	• Whole grain sandwich • Turkey • Avocado • Lettuce	• Cottage cheese • Pineapple	• Grilled fish tacos • Whole grain tortillas • Salsa • Side salad
Sunday	Flex Day Fasting window: 8:00 p.m. (Saturday) to noon Eating window: Noon to 8:00 p.m.	• Flex meal—enjoy a balanced meal of your choice	• Your choice, keeping it balanced and within your nutritional goals	• Balanced meal • Carbs • Protein • Healthy fats

Remember, the key to success is flexibility and listening to your body. It might take some time to find the perfect balance, but with patience and perseverance, you can unlock the full potential of these powerful strategies.

Supplementation for Carb Cycling

Alright, let's get down to one of the most crucial aspects of any effective carb cycling plan: supplementation. Whether you're trying to power through a low-carb day or recover after an intense workout on a high-carb day, the right supplements can make all the difference. They can help you maintain energy levels, support muscle recovery, enhance workout performance, and even stabilize your mood and cognitive function. Let's talk about why these supplements are essential and how you can incorporate them into your carb cycling regimen.

Enhance energy levels: Low-carb days can be particularly challenging because your body is not getting the usual amount of glucose it relies on for energy. This is where supplementation comes into play to ensure you don't feel drained and fatigued.

The B vitamins, particularly B12 and B6, are essential for energy production. They help convert the food you eat into glucose, which gives you the energy to power through your day. On low-carb days, taking a B-complex supplement can help sustain your energy levels and keep you feeling more alert and less fatigued.

Improved Recovery: Recovery is just as important as the workout itself. Your muscles need time to repair and grow stronger, and certain supplements can expedite this process.

After a workout, your muscles are in desperate need of protein to repair the tiny tears that occur during exercise. Whey protein is quickly absorbed by the body, making it an excellent post-workout supplement. It helps in muscle repair and growth, ensuring you're ready for your next workout.

BCAAs are vital for muscle repair and reducing exercise-induced muscle damage. They can also help decrease muscle soreness, allowing you to train harder and more frequently. Taking BCAAs before and after your workouts can significantly enhance your recovery process.

Metabolism Support: A well-functioning metabolism is crucial for effective weight loss and overall health. Certain supplements can support metabolic processes and help your body function optimally.

Omega-3 fatty acids support heart health, reduce inflammation, and can even aid in fat loss. Omega-3s help maintain a healthy metabolic rate, which is crucial when you're trying to lose weight or improve your fitness. They are found in fish oil supplements and are essential for overall well-being.

Enhance Workout Performance: When you're hitting the gym hard, especially on high-carb days, you need all the support you can get to maximize your performance and results.

Creatine is one of the most well-researched supplements out there, known for enhancing strength, muscle mass, and exercise performance. Creatine helps your muscles produce energy during heavy lifting or high-intensity exercise, making it a staple supplement for anyone serious about their workouts.

Coenzyme Q10 (CoQ10) is an antioxidant that plays a critical role in energy production within your cells. It helps improve physical performance and reduce the oxidative stress caused by intense exercise. CoQ10 can also help maintain a healthy heart and blood vessels.

Beta-alanine is an amino acid that helps buffer acid in muscles, increasing physical performance during high-intensity exercise and reducing fatigue. It can help you push through those last few reps, making a significant difference in your workout results.

Stabilize Mood and Cognitive Function: Maintaining a positive mood and sharp cognitive function is crucial, especially when you're adjusting to a new diet and exercise routine. Some supplements can support brain health and help manage stress.

Magnesium is involved in over 300 biochemical reactions in your body, including those that affect muscle function and mood regulation. It can help reduce muscle cramps and improve sleep quality, which is vital for recovery and overall well-being.

Ashwagandha is an adaptogen and is known for its ability to reduce stress and anxiety, improve mood, and enhance overall brain function. It can help you manage the stress that comes with intense training and dietary changes, keeping you calm and focused.

Natural Supplements for Appetite Suppression

When it comes to managing hunger and cravings, natural supplements can be a game-changer. They help control your appetite, making it easier to stick to your diet plan (Vergnaud, 2021).

• **Caralluma fimbriata:** This cactus plant extract is known for its appetite-suppressing properties. It works by increasing the levels of serotonin in your brain, which can reduce hunger and help you feel full faster.

• **Garcinia cambogia plus gymnema sylvestre:** Garcinia cambogia contains hydroxycitric acid (HCA), which helps block fat production and curb appetite. Gymnema sylvestre helps reduce sugar cravings and lower blood sugar levels, making this combination effective for appetite control.

• **5-HTP:** This naturally occurring amino acid is a precursor to serotonin, a neurotransmitter that regulates mood and appetite. Taking 5-HTP can help increase serotonin levels, reduce hunger and cravings, and promote a feeling of fullness.

Detailed Breakdown of Each Supplement

Complex Vitamin B

B vitamins are crucial for energy production and brain function. They help convert the food you eat into energy, keeping you active and alert throughout the day. Take a B-complex supplement in the morning with your first meal to support energy levels throughout the day. This is particularly useful on low-carb days when energy might be low.
Foods rich in Vitamin B: Leafy green vegetables, whole grains, eggs, and meat.

Whey Protein

Whey protein is a complete protein source, meaning it contains all the essential amino acids your body needs. It's quickly absorbed, making it ideal for post-workout recovery. Consume a whey protein shake within 30 minutes post-workout to help repair and build muscle tissue.

Foods rich in Whey Protein: Eggs, chicken breast, fish, and legumes.

Branched Chain Amino Acids (BCAAs)

BCAAs (leucine, isoleucine, and valine) play a critical role in muscle protein synthesis and recovery. They help reduce muscle soreness and fatigue. Take BCAAs before, during, or after your workouts to support muscle recovery and reduce soreness.

Foods rich in BCAAs: Meat, dairy products, and legumes.

Omega-3 Fatty Acids

Omega-3s support heart health, reduce inflammation, and can aid in fat loss. They are essential for maintaining a healthy metabolic rate and overall health. Take an omega-3 supplement daily, ideally with a meal that contains fat, to improve absorption.

Foods rich in Omega-3s: Fatty fish like salmon, walnuts, and flaxseeds.

Creatine

Creatine enhances muscle strength, power, and endurance by increasing the availability of ATP (adenosine triphosphate), the primary energy carrier in cells. Take 3–5 grams of creatine monohydrate daily, ideally post-workout, with a carbohydrate source to improve uptake

Foods rich in Creatine: Red meat and fish.

Coenzyme Q10 (CoQ10)

CoQ10 is essential for energy production in cells and acts as a powerful antioxidant. It helps improve physical performance and reduce exercise-induced oxidative stress. Take 100–200 mg of CoQ10 daily, preferably with a meal that contains fat.
Foods rich in CoQ10: Organ meats, fatty fish, and whole grains.

Beta-Alanine

Beta-alanine increases the concentration of carnosine in muscles, which helps buffer acid and reduce fatigue during high-intensity exercise. Take 2–5 grams of beta-alanine daily, divided into smaller doses to avoid tingling sensations
Foods rich in Beta-Alanine: Poultry, meat, and fish.

Magnesium

Magnesium is crucial for muscle function, mood regulation, and overall health. It helps reduce muscle cramps and improve sleep quality. Take 200–400 mg of magnesium daily, preferably in the evening, to support relaxation and sleep.
Foods rich in Magnesium: Nuts, seeds, leafy greens, and whole grains.

Caralluma Fimbriat

This supplement is known for its appetite-suppressing properties, making it easier to stick to your dietary goals by reducing hunger. Follow the recommended dosage on the supplement packaging, typically taken before meals to help control appetite.
As this is a specific extract, it's not commonly found in everyday foods but can be taken as a supplement.

Garcinia Cambogia Plus Gymnema Sylvestre

Garcinia cambogia helps block fat production and curb appetite, while Gymnema sylvestre reduces sugar cravings and helps control blood sugar levels. Follow the recommended dosage on the supplement packaging, usually taken before meals to maximize its appetite-suppressing effects.

These are primarily found in supplement form rather than in common foods.

5-HTP

5-HTP is a precursor to serotonin, which helps regulate mood and appetite. It can reduce hunger and cravings, making it easier to stick to your diet. Take 100–300 mg of 5-HTP daily, preferably in the evening, to support mood and sleep.

While 5-HTP is typically taken as a supplement, foods rich in tryptophan, like turkey and nuts, can support serotonin production.

Incorporating Supplements into Your Routine

Integrating these supplements into your carb cycling plan can enhance your results and make the process more manageable. Here's how you can effectively incorporate them:

• **Create a supplement schedule:** Plan when to take each supplement based on your daily routine and workout schedule. For example, take whey protein and creatine post-workout, while magnesium can be taken in the evening to aid sleep.

• **Track your progress:** Keep a journal to monitor how you feel after taking each supplement. Note any changes in energy levels, workout performance, recovery, and overall well-being.

• **Consult with a professional:** Before starting any new supplement regimen, it's essential to consult with a healthcare provider or nutritionist to ensure the supplements are appropriate for your needs and won't interact with any medications you're taking.

Supplementation can play a pivotal role in enhancing your carb cycling results. From boosting energy levels and improving recovery to supporting metabolism and stabilizing mood, the right supplements can help you stay on track and achieve your fitness goals.

With advanced strategies in your arsenal, you're now equipped to take your carb cycling to the next level. Whether it's breaking through frustrating plateaus, optimizing your energy and recovery with the right supplements, or understanding the intricate science behind these methods, you've got the knowledge to push forward confidently.

Every journey has its ups and downs, and it's perfectly normal to encounter challenges along the way. The key is to stay informed, be patient with yourself, and remain flexible in your approach. Adjustments are part of the process, and they are often the steps that lead to long-term success.

Think of your journey as climbing a mountain. There will be times when the path is steep and challenging, but with each step, you're getting closer to the peak. Every bit of progress, no matter how small, is a victory. Celebrate these milestones, and use them as motivation to keep moving forward.

The next chapter will guide you through a 7-day diet and exercise plan designed to kickstart your journey. This plan is tailored to help you implement everything you've learned in a structured, practical way, ensuring you start seeing results right away.

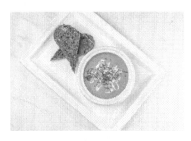

Chapter Eight
7-Day Kickstart Plan

This chapter is where all the theory and strategies we've discussed come together in a practical, actionable format. If you've ever felt overwhelmed by the sheer volume of information about diet and exercise, you're in the right place. This chapter is designed to simplify carb cycling, giving you a structured plan to follow for the next week.

Think of this as your personal roadmap. Over the next seven days, you'll have a clear, step-by-step guide to help you kickstart your carb cycling journey. I've crafted detailed daily meal plans that align with your carb cycling schedule, complete with tips for meal prep to save you time and stress. Each day's plan is tailored to either a high-carb or low-carb day, ensuring you get the right nutrients to fuel your body and maximize fat loss.

It's not just about what you eat. This plan also includes specific daily workout routines designed to complement your carb intake and enhance your results. You'll find guidance on adjusting the intensity of your workouts to match your energy levels, ensuring you stay motivated and avoid burnout. Suitable for both fitness newbies and seasoned pros, these routines can be adapted to fit your fitness level and goals.

Monitoring your progress is crucial, and this chapter provides practical tips on how to track your journey. We'll cover everything from keeping a food journal to taking body measurements and noting changes in how you feel. This isn't just about numbers on a scale—it's about recognizing and celebrating all the small victories along the way.

Starting a new plan can be daunting, but remember, this week is all about setting a strong foundation, learning what works for your body, and making adjustments to optimize your plan. By the end of these seven days, you'll not only see progress but also feel more confident in your ability to manage carb cycling and intermittent fasting.

Tips for Meal Prep and Organization

Let's talk about meal prep and organization because having a solid plan can make all the difference in your success with carb cycling. I've found that dedicating a bit of time each week to plan, shop, and prepare your meals can set you up for a stress-free and effective week of eating right and staying on track. Here's a step-by-step guide to streamline your meal prep process.

Plan Your Meals on Fridays, Shop on Saturdays, and Compile on Sundays

First things first, let's get organized. I recommend setting aside a bit of time each Friday to plan your meals for the upcoming week. This gives you a clear vision of what you'll need, helps you avoid last-minute decisions, and ensures you're sticking to your carb cycling plan. Write down what you'll be eating for breakfast, lunch, dinner, and snacks, and make a comprehensive shopping list.

On Saturdays, take that list and head to the grocery store. Shopping on Saturdays gives you the flexibility to find the best produce and ingredients while avoiding the rush of a Sunday crowd. Plus, it gives you a day to get everything you need without feeling rushed.

Sundays are your meal prep days. This is when you'll put everything together, portion out your meals, and make sure you're ready to tackle the week. Dedicate a couple of hours to cooking, assembling, and storing your meals. Trust me, the effort you put in on Sunday will pay off tenfold during the busy weekdays.

Choose Your Foods Wisely

The key to a successful carb cycling plan is choosing the right foods. Focus on nutrient-dense options that will fuel your body and keep you satisfied.

High-fiber fruits and vegetables: Think berries, apples, broccoli, spinach, and carrots. These foods not only provide essential vitamins and minerals but also keep you feeling full longer.

Low-fat dairy products: Incorporate items like milk, cheese, and yogurt. They're great sources of calcium and protein, which are crucial for muscle maintenance and overall health.

Legumes: Beans, lentils, and peas are fantastic for adding fiber and protein to your meals. They're especially great for low-carb days when you need a filling, nutritious option.

Whole grains: Choose oats, brown rice, quinoa, and whole-wheat products over refined grains. Whole grains provide sustained energy and help keep your blood sugar levels stable.

Restrict refined grains, added sugars, and highly processed foods: These foods can derail your progress by causing blood sugar spikes and contributing to cravings. Stick to whole, unprocessed foods as much as possible.

Use Portion-Controlled Containers

Portion control is critical when you're carb cycling. To make this easier, invest in a set of good-quality, portion-controlled containers. These will help you keep track of your food intake and ensure you're eating the right amounts at each meal.

Here's what I do: After cooking, I divide my meals into these containers, making sure each portion aligns with my high- or low-carb days. For instance, I'll have larger portions of sweet potatoes or brown rice on high-carb days, and more veggies and lean proteins on low-carb days.

Label Each Container

Once your meals are portioned out, label each container clearly. This might seem like a small step, but it makes a big difference. Labeling helps you quickly grab what you need without second-guessing or mixing up your meals.

For breakfast, lunch, dinner, and snacks, use color-coded labels or write directly on the containers with a dry-erase marker. For example, use blue labels for high-carb meals and red labels for low-carb meals. This visual cue simplifies your choices, especially when you're in a hurry.

Meal Prep Steps

Now, let's break down the meal prep process with a detailed plan to ensure you're organized and efficient:

Create a weekly menu: Start by mapping out your week. Note your high- and low-carb days, and plan meals that align with these requirements. Consider your schedule. If you have busy evenings, plan for quick, easy-to-reheat meals on those days.

Make a detailed shopping list: Write down every ingredient you'll need for your meals. Include snacks and condiments to avoid mid-week shopping trips. Check your pantry and fridge before heading out to avoid buying duplicates.

Grocery shopping tips: Stick to your list. It's easy to get sidetracked by tempting, but unnecessary, items. Shop the perimeter of the store. This is where you'll find fresh produce, dairy, and meats. Avoid the aisles where processed foods reside.

Prep like a pro: Start with items that take the longest to cook, like grains and proteins. While they're cooking, you can chop veggies or prepare other components. Cook in batches. For example, roast a large tray of vegetables or cook multiple servings of chicken breasts at once.

Assemble your meals: Once everything is cooked, start assembling your meals. Divide ingredients into your portion-controlled containers. Make sure each meal aligns with your high- or low-carb day. For example, a high-carb lunch might include quinoa, roasted veggies, and grilled chicken. A low-carb dinner might be a big salad with leafy greens, avocado, and a protein like salmon or tofu.

Label and store: Clearly label each container with the meal and day. Use different colors for high-carb and low-carb days to avoid confusion. Store meals in the fridge for easy access. Consider freezing meals if you're prepping more than a week in advance.

Tips for Maintaining Variety

One of the biggest challenges with meal prep is avoiding monotony. Here are some tips to keep things interesting:

• **Rotate ingredients:** Don't eat the same thing every day. Rotate your proteins, veggies, and grains to keep your meals exciting.

• **Experiment with spices and herbs:** These can transform a dish. Keep a variety of spices and herbs on hand to add different flavors to your meals.

• **Try new recipes:** Keep your meal prep exciting by trying new recipes. This keeps things fresh and ensures you're not getting bored with your food.

Staying Flexible

Flexibility is crucial. Life happens, and sometimes plans change. Here's how to stay on track even when things don't go as planned:

Have backup meals: Keep a few easy-to-make options on hand for days when you don't have time to cook. Think frozen veggies, canned beans, and whole grains that cook quickly.

Prep snacks: Healthy snacks can be a lifesaver. Prepare items like cut veggies, hummus, nuts, and fruit to have on hand when hunger strikes.

Meal prep and organization might seem like a lot of work upfront, but it's a game-changer for staying consistent with your carb cycling plan. By dedicating time each week to plan, shop, and prepare your meals, you'll set yourself up for success and reduce stress during the busy weekdays.

7-Day Plan

Let's dive into the nitty-gritty of your 7-day kickstart plan, combining exercise routines with a meal prep strategy tailored to your carb cycling schedule. Having a clear plan for both workouts and meals will not only streamline your week but also ensure you're maximizing your efforts in both areas. Here's how to structure your week for optimal results:

Monday	
Meal Plan: High Carb	
Breakfast	Oatmeal with berries and a spoonful of almond butter
Lunch	Quinoa salad with chickpeas, cucumber, tomatoes, and feta cheese
Dinner	Grilled chicken breast with sweet potato and steamed broccoli
Snacks	Greek yogurt with honey, apple slices with peanut butter
Exercise: HIIT – Upper Body	
Warm-up	5 minutes of light cardio (jogging in place, jumping jacks)
Circuit 1	Push-ups, dumbbell shoulder press, bent over rows (3 sets of 12 reps each)
Circuit 2	Bicep curls, triceps dips, and plank holds (3 sets of 12 reps each)
Cool down	5 minutes of stretching

Tuesday	
Meal Plan: Low Carb	
Breakfast	Scrambled eggs with spinach and mushrooms
Lunch	Mixed greens salad with avocado, grilled chicken, and olive oil dressing
Dinner	Baked salmon with asparagus and a mixed green salad
Snacks	Celery sticks with hummus, mixed nuts
Exercise: Yoga	**60 minutes:** focus on flexibility, balance, and relaxation. Include poses: downward dog, warrior II, and child's pose

Wednesday	
Meal Plan: High Carb	
Breakfast	Whole grain toast with avocado and a poached egg
Lunch	Brown rice bowl with black beans, corn, salsa, and chicken
Dinner	Turkey meatballs with whole grain pasta and marinara sauce
Snacks	Cottage cheese with pineapple, banana with almond butter
Exercise: HIIT – Lower Body	
Warm-up	5 minutes of light cardio (jogging in place, jumping jacks)
Circuit 1	Squats, lunges, deadlifts (3 sets of 12 reps each)
Circuit 2	Step-ups, calf raises, leg press (3 sets of 12 reps each)
Cool down	5 minutes of stretching

Thursday	
Meal Plan: Low Carb	
Breakfast	Greek yogurt with chia seeds and a handful of nuts
Lunch	Tuna salad with mixed greens, cherry tomatoes, and olive oil dressing
Dinner	Grilled shrimp with zucchini noodles and a side salad
Snacks	Bell pepper slices with guacamole, a handful of almonds
Exercise: Hiking or Brisk Walking	**60 minutes:** briskly walk or take a hike in nature. Focus on maintaining a steady pace and enjoying the scenery

Friday	
Meal Plan: Low Carb	
Breakfast	Omelet with bell peppers, onions, and cheese
Lunch	Caesar salad with grilled chicken (light on the dressing)
Dinner	Beef stir-fry with broccoli and cauliflower rice
Snacks	Sliced cucumbers with tzatziki and string cheese
Exercise: Biking (Indoors or Outdoors)	**45 minutes:** steady-state biking, maintaining a moderate pace. Aim for a heart rate that allows you to hold a conversation while still feeling challenged

Saturday	
Meal Plan: High Carb	
Breakfast	Smoothie with spinach, banana, protein powder, and almond milk
Lunch	Chicken and vegetable stir-fry with brown rice
Dinner	Whole-grain pizza with assorted vegetables and lean protein
Snacks	Protein bar, mixed fruit salad
Exercise: HIIT – Total Body Workout	
Warm-up	5 minutes of light cardio (jogging in place, jumping jacks)
Circuit 1	Burpees, jump squats, mountain climbers (3 sets of 12 reps each)
Circuit 2	Kettlebell swings, push-ups, high knees (3 sets of 12 reps each)
Cool down	5 minutes of stretching

Sunday	
Meal Plan: Flex Day	
Breakfast	Protein pancakes with a side of mixed berries
Lunch	Leftover chicken and vegetable stir-fry
Dinner	Grilled fish with a side of roasted vegetables
Snacks	Smoothie with almond milk, spinach, and a scoop of protein powder, trail mix
Exercise: Day Off	**Rest day:** Take a day to allow your body to recover and rejuvenate. Enjoy light activities like walking, stretching, or just relaxing

Modifications for Individuals with Restrictive Motion

Starting a fitness journey can be daunting, especially if you have any physical limitations or restrictive motion. However, it's crucial to remember that exercise is adaptable. The key is to modify workouts to fit your unique needs, ensuring that you can still benefit from physical activity without causing harm or discomfort. Here are some practical tips for adjusting your workouts:

Change Speed to Slow Down: If you find it challenging to keep up with the pace of certain exercises, it's perfectly fine to slow down. Reducing the speed of your movements can help you maintain control and prevent injury. For example, if you're doing a high-intensity interval training (HIIT) workout, you can perform the movements at a slower pace. This allows you to focus on proper form and build strength gradually.

Reduce Impact—Try Exercising in a Pool: High-impact exercises, such as running or jumping, can be tough on your joints. Consider switching to low-impact activities, like swimming or water aerobics. Exercise in a pool provides resistance while significantly reducing the impact on your joints. The buoyancy of the water supports your body weight, making movements easier and more fluid.

Adjust Range of Motion for Your Flexibility and Gradually Increase Over Time: Flexibility varies from person to person, and it's important to work within your current range of motion to avoid strain. Start with smaller, controlled movements and gradually increase your range as your flexibility improves. For instance, if you're doing squats, you can start with shallow squats and slowly progress to deeper ones as your strength and flexibility improve.

Reduce Weight: When lifting weights, it's essential to choose a weight that you can handle comfortably while maintaining proper form. If you find the weights too heavy, reduce the amount of weight you're lifting. Using lighter weights with higher repetitions can still provide an effective workout and help build muscle endurance.

Reduce Number of Repetitions: If doing a full set of repetitions is too challenging, reduce the number of reps. Focus on quality over quantity. Performing fewer repetitions with proper form is more beneficial than completing a full set with poor technique. You can gradually increase the number of repetitions as your strength improves.

Change Your Positioning—Wider Stances or Laying on the Floor: Sometimes, simply adjusting your positioning can make an exercise more manageable. For example, widening your stance during squats or lunges can provide more stability. Similarly, performing exercises on the floor, such as laying down for leg lifts or chest presses, can reduce strain on your joints and back.

Bend Your Elbows and Knees: Bending your elbows and knees slightly during exercises can reduce the strain on your joints. For instance, if you're doing a plank, keep a slight bend in your elbows to take some pressure off your wrists. This adjustment can make exercise more comfortable and sustainable.

Adjust Workout Durations: If you find that longer workouts are too taxing, break them into shorter sessions. Instead of a continuous 45-minute workout, you could do three 15-minute sessions throughout the day. This approach allows you to stay active without overwhelming your body. Listen to your body and rest when needed.

Throughout this chapter, you've learned how to effectively plan and prepare your meals, organize your weekly routine, and incorporate exercises that align with your carb cycling schedule. You've seen how a structured approach can simplify your daily life and ensure you stay on track with your goals. By taking the time to plan your meals on Fridays, shop on Saturdays, and prepare on Sundays, you've set yourself up for success. This level of organization helps eliminate the stress of daily meal decisions and allows you to focus on enjoying your food and workouts.

Looking ahead, it's crucial to remain flexible and adaptable. Life can be unpredictable, and there will be times when things don't go as planned. Whether it's a busy workweek, social commitments, or unexpected events, know that it's okay to adjust your plan. The key is to stay committed to your overall goal and make the best choices possible in any given situation. Adapt your meals, modify your workouts, and always prioritize your well-being.

Afterword

I'm proud of the fact that you've taken a significant step toward transforming your health and fitness through carb cycling. It's been a journey filled with valuable insights, practical tips, and actionable strategies designed to help you succeed.

Let's take a moment to recap everything you've learned:

You started by grasping the fundamentals of carb cycling, learning how alternating between high-carb and low-carb days can optimize metabolism, promote fat loss, and enhance physical performance. You discovered the science behind carbohydrates and their impact on your body, along with the critical role of insulin in weight management.

Chapter by chapter, you learned how to personalize carb cycling for your own lifestyle. Whether your goal is weight loss, muscle gain, or improved athletic performance, you now have the tools to customize your diet and exercise routine accordingly. We also covered how to adapt carb cycling for special diets like vegetarianism and gluten-free lifestyles, ensuring flexibility and sustainability.

Every journey has its hurdles, and we tackled common challenges head-on. You acquired useful techniques to maintain focus, from controlling hunger and urges to interacting with others. I underlined the need for maintaining consistency and motivation and offered advice on how to maintain your momentum even on difficult days.

For those looking to take their carb cycling to the next level, we explored advanced tactics. You now understand how to identify and overcome weight loss plateaus, the benefits of combining intermittent fasting with carb cycling, and how supplementation can enhance your energy, recovery, and overall results.

To set you up for immediate success, I provided a detailed 7-day kickstart plan. This plan included specific daily meal prep tips, exercise routines tailored to high- and low-carb days, and modifications for different fitness levels. By following this structured approach, you can begin your carb cycling journey with confidence.

With all this knowledge at your fingertips, you're well-equipped to embark on your carb cycling journey. The most important thing now is to take action. Remember, the information you've gained is powerful, but it's the implementation that will drive your transformation. Here's your call to action:

• Use the 7-day kickstart plan as your guide, and don't be afraid to make adjustments based on your personal preferences and needs. Stay committed to your goals, be patient with yourself, and celebrate every milestone along the way.

• Set specific, attainable goals, and push yourself to achieve them. Whether it's completing a full week of carb cycling, hitting a new personal best in your workouts, or mastering a healthy meal prep routine, each challenge you overcome will build your confidence and momentum.

• Share your journey with friends, family, or even on social media. By doing so, you not only hold yourself accountable but also inspire those around you to take charge of their health. Who knows, you might find a workout buddy or a meal prep partner along the way!

• Life is unpredictable, and there will be times when things don't go as planned. That's okay. Adjust your approach as needed, and always prioritize your well-being. Remember, this is a marathon, not a sprint.

Now, armed with all the knowledge and strategies from this book, it's time to put it into practice. Embrace the process, enjoy the journey, and watch as you transform into a healthier, stronger version of yourself. So, go out there and make it happen!

Bibliography

1. Bayham, B. E., Greenway, F. L., Johnson, W. D., & Dhurand-har, N. V. (2014). A randomized trial to manipulate the quality instead of quantity of dietary proteins to influence the markers of satiety. *Journal of Diabetes and Its Complications, 28*(4), 547–552. https://doi.org/10.1016/j.jdiacomp.2014.02.002

2. *Carb cycling 101: Benefits and how to get started.* (n.d.). Carb Manager. Retrieved May 18, 2024, from https://www.carbmanager.com/article/zumbzhyaacqabt eg/carb-cycling-101-benefits-and-how-to-get-started

3. Cherney, K. (2023, May 10). *Simple carbohydrates vs. complex carbohydrates.* Healthline. https://www.healthline.com/health /food-nutrition/simple-carbohydrates-complex-carbohydrates

4. *Carbohydrates.* (2021, February 8). Cleveland Clinic. https://m y.clevelandclinic.org/health/articles/15416-carbohydrates

5. Corney, R. A., Sunderland, C., & James, L. J. (2015). Immediate pre-meal water ingestion decreases voluntary food intake in lean young males. *European Journal of Nutrition, 55*(2), 815–819. ht tps://doi.org/10.1007/s00394-015-0903-4

6. Cronkleton , E. (2022, April 29). *6 ways to bust through a workout plateau.* Healthline. https://www.healthline.com/nut rition/workout-plateau

7. Deota, S., Lin, T., Chaix, A., Williams, A., Le, H., Calligaro, H., Ramasamy, R., Huang, L., & Panda, S. (2023). Diurnal

transcriptome landscape of a multi-tissue response to time-restricted feeding in mammals. *Cell Metabolism, 35*(1), 150-165.e4. https://doi.org/10.1016/j.cmet.2022.12.006

8. DiLonardo, M. J. (2022, August 8). *Carb cycling.* WebMD. https://www.webmd.com/diet/carb-cycling-overview

9. Garnet health. (2016, July 1). *Basal metabolic rate calculator.* Garnet Health. https://www.garnethealth.org/news/basal-metabolic-rate-calculator

10. Gunnars, K. (2018, December 4). *Leptin and leptin resistance: Everything you need to know.* Healthline. https://www.healthline.com/nutrition/leptin-101

11. Gunnars, K. (2023, October 31). *What is intermittent fasting and how does it work?* Healthline. https://www.healthline.com/nutrition/10-health-benefits-of-intermittent-fasting

12. Gunnars, K. (2024, May 3). *Intermittent fasting 101 — the ultimate beginner's guide.* Healthline. https://www.healthline.com/nutrition/intermittent-fasting-guide

13. Hansen, T. T., Astrup, A., & Sjödin, A. (2021). Are dietary proteins the key to successful body weight management? A systematic review and meta-analysis of studies assessing body weight outcomes after interventions with increased dietary protein. *Nutrients, 13*(9), 3193. https://doi.org/10.3390/nu13093193

14. Harvard Health Publishing. (2021, April 19). *Know the facts about fats.* Harvard Health. https://www.health.harvard.edu/staying-healthy/know-the-facts-about-fats

15. Haseltine, W. A. (2023, February 10). *Can intermittent fasting help you live longer?* Forbes. https://www.forbes.com/sites/williamhaseltine/2023/02/10/can-intermittent-fasting-help-you-live-longer/

16. Holesh, J. E., Martin, A., & Aslam, S. (2023, May 12). *Physiology,*

Carbohydrates. Nih.gov; StatPearls Publishing. https://www.n cbi.nlm.nih.gov/books/NBK459280/

17. Hollis, J. F., Gullion, C. M., Stevens, V. J., Brantley, P. J., Appel, L. J., Ard, J. D., Champagne, C. M., Dalcin, A., Erlinger, T. P., Funk, K., Laferriere, D., Lin, P.-H., Loria, C. M., Samuel-Hodge, C., Vollmer, W. M., & Svetkey, L. P. (2008). Weight loss during the intensive intervention phase of the weight-loss maintenance trial. *American Journal of Preventive Medicine, 35*(2), 118–126. https://doi.org/10.1016/j.amepre.2008.04.013

18. Kandola, A., & French, M. (2023, November 29). *What are the benefits of intermittent fasting?* Www.medicalnewstoday.com. https://www.medicalnewstoday.com/articles/323605

19. Kubala, J. (2018, October 14). *How to count macros: A step-by-step guide.* Healthline. https://www.healthline.com/n utrition/how-to-count-macros

20. Li, S. S., Kendall, C. W. C., de Souza, R. J., Jayalath, V. H., Cozma, A. I., Ha, V., Mirrahimi, A., Chiavaroli, L., Augustin, L. S. A., Blanco Mejia, S., Leiter, L. A., Beyene, J., Jenkins, D. J. A., & Sievenpiper, J. L. (2014). Dietary pulses, satiety and food intake: A systematic review and meta-analysis of acute feeding trials. *Obesity, 22*(8), 1773–1780. https://doi.org/10.1002/oby.2 0782

21. Lindberg, S. (2019, October 3). *LISS cardio: Benefits vs. HIIT, heart rate, workout.* Healthline. https://www.healthline.com/ health/exercise-fitness/liss-cardio

22. Link, R. (2023, October 27). *Glycemic index: What it is and how to use it.* Healthline. https://www.healthline.com/nutrition/gl ycemic-index

23. Mandolesi, L., Polverino, A., Montuori, S., Foti, F., Ferraioli, G., Sorrentino, P., & Sorrentino, G. (2018). Effects of physical exercise on cognitive functioning and wellbeing: Biological and

psychological benefits. *Frontiers in Psychology*, *9*(9). https://d oi.org/10.3389/fpsyg.2018.00509

24. Martins, N. (2019, November 10). *Carb cycling guide for athletes.* Ketone-IQ®. https://ketone.com/blogs/blog/training-carb-cycl ing-guide-for-athletes

25. Mawer, R. (2023, March 20). *11 ways to boost human growth hormone (HGH) naturally.* Healthline; Healthline Media. htt ps://www.healthline.com/nutrition/11-ways-to-increase-hgh

26. Mayo Clinic Staff. (2021, October 8). *7 great reasons why exercise matters.* Mayo Clinic; Mayo Foundation for Medical Education and Research. https://www.mayoclinic.org/healthy-lifestyle/fit ness/in-depth/exercise/art-20048389

27. McCrickerd, K., & Forde, C. (2017). Consistency of eating rate, oral processing behaviours and energy intake across meals. *Nu-trients*, *9*(8), 891. https://doi.org/10.3390/nu9080891

28. McNeil, J., Cadieux, S., Finlayson, G., Blundell, J. E., & Doucet, É. (2015). The effects of a single bout of aerobic or resistance exercise on food reward. *Appetite*, *84*, 264–270. https://doi.o rg/10.1016/j.appet.2014.10.018

29. *Mifflin-St Jeor equation.* (2020). Reference.medscape.com . https://reference.medscape.com/calculator/846/mifflin-st-jeo r-equation

30. Mitchell, L., Hackett, D., Gifford, J., Estermann, F., & O'Con-nor, H. (2017). Do bodybuilders use evidence-based nutrition strategies to manipulate physique? *Sports*, *5*(4). https://doi.or g/10.3390/sports5040076

31. Nesterova, A. P., Klimov, E. A., Zharkova, M., Sozin, S., Sobolev, V., Ivanikova, N. V., Shkrob, M., & Yuryev, A. (2020). En-docrine, nutritional, and metabolic diseases. *Disease Pathways*, 121–218. https://doi.org/10.1016/b978-0-12-817086-1.00004-x

32. Pearson, K. (2017, November 9). *What are the key functions of carbohydrates?* Healthline. https://www.healthline.com/nutrition/carbohydrate-functions

33. Peos, J., Norton, L., Helms, E., Galpin, A., & Fournier, P. (2019). Intermittent dieting: Theoretical considerations for the athlete. *Sports, 7*(1), 22. https://doi.org/10.3390/sports7010022

34. Phelps, N. (2019, March 29). *What is BMR and TDEE + how to use them to lose weight.* Chomps. https://chomps.com/blogs/nutrition-sustainability-news/what-is-bmr-tdee

35. *Physical activity guidelines for Americans.* (2018, November 12). HHS.gov. https://www.hhs.gov/fitness/be-active/physical-activity-guidelines-for-americans/index.html

36. Reed, G. W., & Hill, J. O. (1996). Measuring the thermic effect of food. *The American Journal of Clinical Nutrition, 63*(2), 164–169. https://doi.org/10.1093/ajcn/63.2.164

37. Rolls, B. J. (2017). Dietary energy density: Applying behavioural science to weight management. *Nutrition Bulletin, 42*(3), 246–253. https://doi.org/10.1111/nbu.12280

38. Sharafi, M., Alamdari, N., Wilson, M., Leidy, H. J., & Glynn, E. L. (2018). Effect of a high-protein, high-fiber beverage preload on subjective appetite ratings and subsequent ad libitum energy intake in overweight men and women: A randomized, double-blind placebo-controlled, crossover study. *Current Developments in Nutrition, 2*(6). https://doi.org/10.1093/cdn/nzy022

39. Slyper, A. (2021). Oral processing, satiation and obesity: Overview and hypotheses. *Diabetes, Metabolic Syndrome and Obesity: Targets and Therapy, Volume 14*, 3399–3415. https://doi.org/10.2147/dmso.s314379

40. Snyder, C., & Gunnars, K. (2023, June 21). *Pros and cons of 5 intermittent fasting methods.* Healthline. https://www.healthl

ine.com/nutrition/6-ways-to-do-intermittent-fasting

41. Tinsley, G. (2017, June 2). *7 benefits of high-intensity interval training (HIIT)*. Healthline; Healthline Media. https://www.healthline.com/nutrition/benefits-of-hiit

42. Van De Walle, G. (2023, February 15). *9 important functions of protein in your body*. Healthline. https://www.healthline.com/nutrition/functions-of-protein

43. Vergnaud, S. (2021, March 24). *Natural appetite suppressants: What to know*. GoodRx; GoodRx. https://www.goodrx.com/well-being/diet-nutrition/best-natural-appetite-suppressants

44. Washington, N. (2022, April 20). *How exercise can help manage stress, anxiety, and depression*. Www.medicalnewstoday.com. https://www.medicalnewstoday.com/articles/how-does-exercise-reduce-stress

45. Yang, C.-L., Schnepp, J., & Tucker, R. M. (2019). Increased hunger, food cravings, food reward, and portion size selection after sleep curtailment in women without obesity. *Nutrients*, *11*(3). https://doi.org/10.3390/nu11030663

46. Yuan, X., Wang, J., Yang, S., Gao, M., Cao, L., Li, X., Hong, D., Tian, S., & Sun, C. (2022). Effect of intermittent fasting diet on glucose and lipid metabolism and insulin resistance in patients with impaired glucose and lipid metabolism: A systematic review and meta-analysis. *International Journal of Endocrinology*, *2022*, 1–9. https://doi.org/10.1155/2022/6999907

47. Zambon, V. (2021, March 31). *Carb cycling: Benefits, evidence, and how to do it*. Www.medicalnewstoday.com. https://www.medicalnewstoday.com/articles/carb-cycling

Image References

1. Borba, J. (2019, October 14). *Woman doing sit ups* [Image]. Pex-

els. https://www.pexels.com/photo/woman-doing-sit-ups-307 6516/

2. Cats Coming. (2019, September 15). *Round white ceramic bowl with rice* [Image]. Pexels. https://www.pexels.com/photo/rou nd-white-ceramic-bowl-with-rice-2942320/

3. Cowley, N. (2018, June 11). *Woman holding gray steel spoon* [Image]. Pexels. https://www.pexels.com/photo/woman-hold ing-gray-steel-spoon-1153370/

4. Demidov, A. (2022, May 27). *Close up photo of acai bowl* [Image]. Pexels. https://www.pexels.com/photo/close-up-photo-o f-acai-bowl-12273052/

5. Fotios, L. (2018, June 14). *Assorted fruits on plate* [Image]. Pexels. https://www.pexels.com/photo/assorted-fruits-on-plat e-1161682/

6. Gromov, D. (2021, May 4). *Close-up shot of soup* [Image]. Pexels. https://www.pexels.com/photo/close-up-shot-of-soup-in-a -bowl-beside-a-bread-7780033/

7. Hamra, J. (2018, August 7). *Egg near blueberries* [Image]. Pexels. https://www.pexels.com/photo/egg-near-blueberries-1305063/

8. Makafood. (2021, July 24). *Close-up shot of a pasta* [Image]. Pexels. https://www.pexels.com/photo/close-up-shot-of-a-past a-on-a-plate-8886627/

9. Mirandilla, N. (2019, November 6). *Cooked food on plate* [Image]. Pexels. https://www.pexels.com/photo/photo-of-cooked -food-on-plate-3186649/

10. Olsson, E. (2018, November 28). *Vegetable salad in bowls* [Image]. Pexels. https://www.pexels.com/photo/photo-of-vegetab le-salad-in-bowls-1640770/

Would love your feedback!

Enjoyed reading *The Ultimate Guide to Carb Cycling for Beginners*? We'd love to hear your thoughts! Scan the QR code and leave your feedback on Amazon—your review helps us improve and reach more readers like you! Thank you for your support!

Made in the USA
Columbia, SC
25 May 2025

58443198R00076